MEDICAL
EDUCATION

A History in 100 Images

MEDICAL EDUCATION

A History in 100 Images

Kieran Walsh
Clinical Director of Clinical Improvement
BMJ Learning and Quality
London, UK

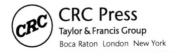

CRC Press
Taylor & Francis Group
Boca Raton London New York

CRC Press is an imprint of the
Taylor & Francis Group, an **informa** business

Acknowledgement: Images courtesy of the Wellcome Library, London, with kind permission.

Image copyrights remain with the individual holders, primarily but not exclusively The Wellcome Trust.

CRC Press
Taylor & Francis Group
6000 Broken Sound Parkway NW, Suite 300
Boca Raton, FL 33487-2742

Printed on acid-free paper
Version Date: 20160414

International Standard Book Number-13: 978-1-4987-5196-4 (Paperback)

Visit the Taylor & Francis Web site at
http://www.taylorandfrancis.com

and the CRC Press Web site at
http://www.crcpress.com

To Sarah Jane, Tommie Jack and Catie Sue, without whom this book would not have been written.

CONTENTS

CONTENTS

FOREWORD

The education of medical students has an impressive lineage spanning many thousands of years. During this time, it has expanded to become a vast educational system incorporating numerous universities, hospitals and clinics spread across the globe. Over the years, medical education has inevitably witnessed a range of shifts in learning and teaching. For example, we have seen the field evolve from a largely didactic endeavour where students were regarded as 'empty vessels' that needed filling with medical knowledge and clinical skills to one which is more mindful and emphasises active engagement with the learners. Similarly, we have seen its curricula evolve from aiming to produce individuals who practice medicine as a solo activity to those who aim to produce practitioners with a range of medical, ethical and collaborative competencies. With the recent centenary of the Flexner Report that resulted in a significant reform of medical education across North America, the historical antecedents of medical education have been brought back into focus. The publication of this book therefore is very timely as it offers an illuminating insight into how the education of medical students has evolved over thousands of years.

On one level, the book's 100 images offer a rich visual account of the various facets to medical education over the years: the contributions of thought leaders, the development of medical equipment and clinical techniques and the creation of new teaching and learning spaces. However, the book also generates a number of underlying issues linked to the development of medical education.

Collectively, the images in the book reinforced the notion of *maleness* of medical education. While we are now seeing more women entering medicine, the roots of the profession are almost exclusively male. As the pictures show, virtually all the notable medical educators (and their students) were men. Women can be found in the book. Elizabeth Garrett Anderson (Image 67) and Sophia Jex-Blake (Image 71) were both influential in advancing medical education for women. In direct contrast to these women and their contributions, the only other prominent female image is more passive in nature – a wax anatomical figure of a partially dissected reclining woman (Image 46), which has a strangely haunting quality to it – like John Everett Millais' painting of the dead Ophelia.

A number of the pictures in the book also suggest the imbalanced relationship that existed between medical educators and patients. Specifically, one can see how passive patients were, as shown in dissections or examinations or the medical education activities of teachers and students. Examples can be found in Image 39 which shows a group of doctors and medical students surrounding a dying patient and Image 93 where a crowd of medical staff stand around a woman patient in bed in a hospital ward. This passivity of the patient's body and, therefore, its objectification in relation to medicine was something that Michael Foucault (1) expressed so effectively in his notion of the *medical gaze* (a term to denote the dehumanizing medical separation of the patient's body from their identity). One can clearly see this in a number of images of medical education through the ages.

The pictures of John Banester giving the visceral lecture at the Barber-Surgeons' Hall (Image 26) and Ambroise Paré at work in his barber-surgeon shop in Paris (Image 24) serve as a useful reminder of the origins of modern Western medicine. Looking at both pictures one sees how, for example, the origins of surgery lay in the work of barbers – tradesmen (for there were only men involved) – who performed clinical procedures without any formal education. Surgery was initially a self-taught activity: skills were developed on the job in barber shops and were then passed on to their apprentices. While the apprentice model continues to exist in medical education, thankfully the science and evidence base for clinical procedures have vastly improved.

There is a *theatrical* element to many of these pictures. As displayed in a number of the images, the use of operating theatres (with captive audiences of medical students watching a dissection) was widespread. Connected to this idea of audience, it is striking how many pictures show how observation was employed as a key method of learning.

Finally, it is intriguing that nearly all the pictures in the book are formal in nature: staged and posed images of lectures, examinations, ceremonies and portraits. Collectively, these images offer a specific insight into medical education – its 'front stage'. While there is a rich array of images related to the varying elements of educating medical students, in general they only offer a *purposefully posed* history. As a result, what we do not see in these images is the informal (backstage) elements of medical education (sometimes referred to as the hidden curriculum) so well described by Becker (2) and Sinclair (3), in which students' hidden games, rituals and interactions are played out.

Overall, this book provides a striking collection of images that offers an absorbing overview of the evolution of medical education – from the third millennium BC with an image of Shen Nung, the father of Chinese medicine, to William Harvey demonstrating his theory of circulation of the blood in the 1600s, to an Eagle Simulator used to train students at the Chelsea and Westminster Hospital in 2000. This set of historical images captures an essence of the advancement of medical education, and, as such, it provides a stimulating and thought-provoking text.

Professor Scott Reeves
Kingston University & St George's University of London
London, United Kingdom

References

1. Foucault M. *The Birth of the Clinic: An Archaeology of Medical Perception*. Penguin: London, UK, 1973.

2. Becker H, Geer B, Hughes E, Strauss A. *Boys in White: Student Culture in Medical Education*. University of Chicago Press: Chicago, IL, 1961.

3. Sinclair S. *Making Doctors: An Institutional Apprenticeship*. Berg: Oxford, UK, 1997.

PREFACE

Medical education is important. It is important for patients and the public that we have adequate numbers of high-quality medical professionals – and this is only possible by means of high-quality medical education. Medical education has undergone a period of rapid reform over the past 30 years, and yet reform did not start in the 1980s or even the 1880s. Reform of medical education has been around as long as medical education has been around. It can come as a shock to the newcomer that John Shaw Billings was promoting continuous professional development over 100 years ago, that Vesalius was encouraging the active role of the learner over 400 years ago and that Huang Ti and Ch'i Po used questions and answers to engage learners over 4000 years ago. The lesson is clear: we can learn a lot from the past. The purpose of this short book is to introduce the newcomer to the history of medical education and to share some of the lessons that I have learned.

This is a short book and it is impossible to give a comprehensive account of the history of medical education in 100 images. I have had to make choices and ultimately to stop choosing. Inevitably significant figures in medical education have been omitted as, no doubt, have many innovations. Nonetheless, I hope that many important images have been included and that the book gives a helpful introduction to the subject. I have also done my best to include images that engage and entertain as well as educate. You can study assessment methods for licentiates in the eighteenth century, and yet no text will capture the confusion and chaos of Roderick Random's examination – with examiners so engrossed in argument that they ignore the candidate. You can read about the history of education in professionalism, but a picture of a medical student using *Quain's Anatomy* as a beer mat is likely to be much more memorable. The target audience of the book is largely those with an interest in medical education. Academic medical education historians may find it of interest, but the core audience is physicians, medical teachers, students and educationalists. As such, much of the text deliberately relates the image back to its relevance in medical education today.

I have been fortunate in finding such a generous and comprehensive source in Wellcome Images. Wellcome Images has done a service to generations of students of medical education and medicine more generally by putting their catalogue online and making such a rich resource freely available. For 5 years I have thought about this book and wondered if it was possible, and it is mainly thanks to Wellcome Images that the idea has become reality. Particularly, thanks go to Miriam Ward for her time and advice. My colleagues at BMJ, Edward Briffa and Catrin Thomas, also deserve special mention for their encouragement and support.

The images are from Wellcome but the accompanying text is my own. It has been a pleasure to read about the history of medical education from a variety of sources, and I have learned a great deal in the process. I have done my best to ensure that the historical detail in the text is correct; however, if there are any failures in accuracy, then they are my own.

The interested reader will also spend time wondering why some of these images were created, who were the people who created them and what the images meant to their creators. Sometimes answers to these questions will be clear but often they will not be. What is certain, however, is that all of these images were created for a purpose – and sometimes a political or rhetorical purpose. The images are more than just direct reproductions of figures or events from the past. The creator of the image has often made a deliberate choice to portray things in a certain way. Reflecting on why the creator might have done this can often shed as much light on past ideas about medical education as the images themselves. Where possible, I have articulated such reflections in the accompanying text; however, the insightful viewer will often formulate their own thoughts.

This book has been written in three phases. The first phase was easy – searching for images and researching their content. The second phase involved deciding which images would make it into the chosen hundred – and that was harder. For some historical figures, there are a range of images to choose from – which should I pick? Ultimately, I chose those that capture the essence of the person or that show them in action. So Thomas Henry Huxley (nicknamed Darwin's bulldog for his aggressive defence of Darwin's ideas) is portrayed in typically forthright pose. And of course Osler is pictured at the bedside. The final phase was putting the images together and explaining their historical context and/or relevance for today. Sequencing the photographs in a chronological order seemed to be simplest and most logical. In addition to spanning the ages, I have tried to create a book that spans the continents. Many of the images are European in origin, but significant numbers have been deliberately chosen from North America, Asia, the Middle East and Africa. Many regions have a story to tell in the history of medical education.

As the project drew to a close, people inevitably started to ask me what my favourite image was. My favourite is 'The Anatomy Lesson of Dr. Nicolaes Tulp' (Image 31). Tulp was a Dutch surgeon and was to be immortalised by Rembrandt in this painting. The image brings to mind Bagehot's comment on history:

> The best history is but like the art of Rembrandt; it casts a vivid light on certain selected causes, on those which were best and greatest; it leaves all the rest in shadow and unseen. (1)

Dr Kieran Walsh

Reference

1. Bagehot W, *Physics and Politics* (1872), Ch. 2, Sect. 2, Twayne Publishers.

ACKNOWLEDGEMENTS

We thank Wellcome Library, London, for permission to use images from its collection in this book.

AUTHOR

Dr Kieran Walsh is clinical director of Clinical Improvement at BMJ, London, United Kingdom. He is responsible for the editorial direction of its resources in medical education, quality improvement and evidence-based medicine. He has written more than 200 articles for publication – mainly in the field of medical education. He has written three books – *Cost Effectiveness in Medical Education*, *Medical Education: A Dictionary of Quotations* and the *Oxford Textbook of Medical Education*. He has worked in the past as a hospital doctor, specialising in care of the elderly medicine and neurology.

INTRODUCTION

What drives history? Is it politics or policy? Economics or epidemiology? Industry or ideas? Or could it simply be people? *Another Day of Life* by Ryszard Kapuściński tells the story of the Angolan Civil War. At a turning point in the war, one of the factions – the People's Movement for the Liberation of Angola (MPLA) – controlled the capital and the opposing faction controlled the surrounding countryside. Kapuściński describes the reliance of the MPLA on two individuals: a pilot who flies their only plane and an engineer who supplies water to the city. If either of them is killed, the war will be over. This is just one example of individuals having an enormous influence on events. As de Bellaigue writes, 'so much for the inevitability of history' (1).

The history of medicine and of medical education is similarly a history of people. Great ideas, developments and theories loom large – but great individuals tower over them. It is impossible to imagine the history of education in the clinical method without William Osler or the history of curriculum reform without Abraham Flexner. Indeed, the big four of Johns Hopkins Hospital (William Osler, William Welch, William Halsted and Howard Atwood Kelly) were to dominate medical education for most of the twentieth century. It works the other way too – Boerhaave cannot and should not be extricated from the historical context of the Dutch Golden Age. Claude Bernard cannot be described without reference to the reforms of the nineteenth century. For this reason, this history is foremost a history of people and the challenges that they faced and the ideas they developed to overcome these challenges.

The first years of the twenty-first century are certainly a time of both change and challenge in medical education. Multiple forces from multiple sources are pushing medicine and medical education in a variety of different directions. An ageing population with multiple co-morbidities means that we need different types of healthcare professionals to those which we needed in the past. More people with chronic diseases who know more about their health than ever before and want to be a partner in their disease management similarly has changed the role of the healthcare professional. At the same time, the need to improve quality, ensure patient safety and control costs means that healthcare professionals need to have different skills to those which they have had in the past. And also at the same time we face a knowledge explosion and a technology explosion. Today, there is more scientific knowledge than ever before – making it impossible for an individual to learn everything about medicine. Simultaneously, advances in technology mean that anyone has the means of accessing that knowledge – the medical library is now open to everyone.

This perfect storm of changes in medicine will mean changes for medical education. Is it changing fast enough? Or it is still stuck in the models of the last century? Does medical education now concentrate more on primary care than on tertiary care? Is medical education now on the ground or still in the ivory tower? Is it interdisciplinary or uniprofessional? Most importantly, is medical education aligned with healthcare workforce and population needs? If it is not, then we are spending time, funds and resources and yet failing to produce healthcare professionals that the population needs. There needs to be alignment between the skills of the medical workforce and population needs – and modern medical education will need to ensure that this alignment happens (2).

For all this to happen, medical education will have to change. How should it decide how to change? Should it conduct trials of different educational methods and discover what works best? Should it look to big data and conduct large-scale, long-term, real-world studies based on this data? Should it conduct more qualitative research to find out how different educational interventions work? It might need to do many of these things, but all forms of research should start with a look back at what has been done before. Today, we call this process a systematic review – but it has always been with us. Isaac Newton called it 'standing on the shoulders of giants'. The temptation for the modern medical educator is to start with a *tabula rasa* – to think that the problems we face today are so different to those of the past that there is no point in looking back. This is a temptation that should be resisted. There is no question that we can learn from the past and that the problems of the past find resonance with our problems today. Just one example is Sir Thomas Clifford Allbutt worrying about curriculum overload over 100 years ago (3). And there is also no question that the medical education leaders of today can learn from the leaders of yesteryear. Better still that they can find inspiration from them.

The history of medical education has no clear beginning and so it is fitting that this book should start in prehistory. The first image is that of a statue of Asclepius, the Greek god of medicine and healing. The Greeks had multiple gods – from Aphrodite to Zeus – and a range of titans, heroes, kings and deified mortals. Medicine was sufficiently important to warrant its own deity; and this was to echo down the ages in a variety of ways – both for better and for worse. Patients have always wanted physicians who were wise, noble and strong – as Asclepius was. But in the modern era, we no longer want physicians with a sense of infallibility or overweening privilege. And yet the physician-as-god phenomenon has shown remarkable persistence. During my research for this book, the number of leading medical educators who were to be bestowed with the title 'father of' was surprising. So there is a father of medicine, a father of paediatrics, a father of obstetrics – the list goes on. Indeed, many vie for the title of father of surgery – these include Susruta, Guy de Chauliac, Ambroise Paré and Joseph Lister. What does this say about medicine and medical education? Critics would say that it suggests paternalism, attitudes of superiority, or a feeling that patients or learners can be treated like children.

However, one undoubted benefit of having Asclepius is that it gave physicians a god to swear to. Thus, the Hippocratic Oath starts, 'I swear by Apollo the physician, and Asclepius the surgeon, likewise Hygeia and Panacea, and call all the gods and goddesses to witness, that I will observe and keep this underwritten oath, to the utmost of my power and judgment.' (4) The Greeks were to have a strong influence on medicine and medical education, and Hippocrates led the way. He wrote extensively on medical education: 'Instruction in medicine is like the culture of the productions of the earth. For our natural disposition, is, as it were, the soil; the tenets of our teacher are, as it were, the seed; instruction in youth is like the planting of the seed in the ground at the proper season; the place where the instruction is communicated is like the food imparted to vegetables by the atmosphere; diligent study is like the cultivation of the fields; and it is time which imparts strength to all things and brings them to maturity.' (5) Hippocrates is also clear that medical education must continue throughout the physician's life and that instruction is no replacement for experience: 'Having brought all these requisites to the study of medicine, and having acquired a true knowledge of it, we shall thus, in travelling through the cities, be esteemed physicians not only in name but in reality. But inexperience is a bad treasure, and a bad fund to those who possess it, whether in opinion or reality, being devoid of self-reliance and contentedness, and the nurse both of timidity and audacity. For timidity betrays a want of powers, and audacity a lack of skill.' (5) In parallel with Western traditions, medical education was also developing in China, Egypt and India. All can claim to have had a pivotal influence on the earliest development of medical education.

The ancients were to have a long influence on medical education – indeed some would say that their influence lasted too long. Many of their ideas – right or wrong – were to remain unchallenged for centuries. However, challenge did eventually come – starting with the Renaissance. Thomas Linacre was to change learning in medicine in the United Kingdom after returning to London fresh with ideas from Italy. His influence continues today in the Royal College Physicians which he founded.

The experimental method was also to have a transformational impact on medicine and medical education. One early proponent of this method was Ambroise Paré – a French military barber-surgeon who compared different treatments on different groups of patients. New researchers started to overturn the ideas of the ancient scholars – Vesalius, for example, disproved some of the teachings of Galen. Once such new thinking started, it was impossible to stop, and not even a generation was to pass before Realdo Colombo was to challenge the ideas of Vesalius. Medicine and medical education were entering a stage of flux.

Knowledge was subsequently to grow rapidly throughout the seventeenth and eighteenth centuries. William Harvey revolutionised medical thinking with his treatise *On the Motion of the Heart and Blood in Animals*. However, Harvey was more than just a researcher – he was also a keen educator and lectured tirelessly on his discoveries. Another of the great powerhouses of medical education in this epoch was Boerhaave. According to Hull, 'as a master of bedside teaching Boerhaave can be regarded as the originator of modern medical education.' (6) Such was Boerhaave's popularity at the University of Leiden that more space had to be provided to accommodate his students – indeed, places had to be reserved in advance. Learners from around the world would travel to hear Boerhaave – a tradition of medical pilgrimage to places of learning that continues to this day. Many of his students subsequently returned to their home countries and founded or became leading lights in medical schools around the world – from Ireland in the Old World to Philadelphia in the New World. Boerhaave did little original research and is largely remembered for his teaching activities. At a time when medical schools are attempting to rebalance their teaching and research activities, Boerhaave remains an exemplar of how education should be at the core of a medical school's activities.

The nineteenth century was to be one of reform. And the reformers were keen on improving science, medicine and medical education. Oliver Wendell Holmes was an American physician, educator and author. Like many other nineteenth-century reformers, he realised that infection was often caused by poor hygiene, and he was keen to use medical education as a means to disseminate new knowledge in this field. Ignaz Philipp Semmelweis discovered that antiseptic procedures could markedly reduce the occurrence of puerperal fever and save mothers' lives. But his findings were rejected by the medical establishment and he died in an asylum in 1865. However, towards the end of the century what had seemed like heresy was accepted as scientific fact. Joseph Lister introduced antiseptic surgery to the United Kingdom – his championing of such ideas helped them to become mainstream.

The reform of the nineteenth century was to lead to revolution in the twentieth. William Osler and Abraham Flexner were giants in the twentieth-century medical education and their ideas were to have an enormous influence on how medical education was delivered. Osler introduced the concept of the clinical clerkship for undergraduates – whereby senior medical students spent time on the wards taking histories, conducting examinations and following up patients. He also established residencies for doctors in training. Abraham Flexner was an American educationalist who is most famous for the Flexner report. This report made recommendations regarding the provision of medical education in medical schools in the United States. The report drove up standards in medical schools by increasing the requirements needed by entrants, by insisting that physicians receive proper training in medicine as a science and by ensuring that faculty engaged in research and teaching. To close the circle, Flexner held up Osler's Johns Hopkins Hospital as the ideal that medical education institutions should aspire to.

It is impossible to touch on all the historical chapters in medical education in this short introduction. Another perspective on the content can be achieved by way of examining themes. One important theme in the history of medical education is the education of women as physicians. Some would say that for many years this was a theme that was most significant by its absence. Until the modern era, women were denied the opportunity to train as physicians. However, one surprising figure that emerges from the ancient texts is that of Trotula. By some accounts, Trotula was a female Italian gynaecologist and educator at the medical school in Salerno. However, there is uncertainty as to whether she is a historical figure or a mythical one. But there is no doubt as to the existence of the formidable Elizabeth Garret Anderson and to the history that she was to make. Garrett Anderson was the first woman in Britain to qualify as a physician. Her story is one of determination, struggle and eventual triumph against the medical authorities. In addition to being the first female physician in Britain she was also the first female member of the British Medical Association. She was to remain the only female member for 19 years as the association moved to block other women from joining. Today the majority of students at medical school in the United Kingdom are female.

Assessment and examinations always loom large in any text on medical education and this book is no different. Assessment is a dominant theme in medical education discourse mainly because of the effect that it has on learning. Medical students and postgraduate learners know that they must pass exams to progress and so will spend their time studying to help pass these exams. So if exams test recall of scientific knowledge, then that is what learners will concentrate on. The same is true if exams test medical rarities or ephemera. Unfortunately, in the past, examinations often did test these very things. So many of the images in the book show candidates being alternatively humiliated, tortured or ignored by their examiners. Regrettably, some of them are from the recent past. Hopefully they will serve as a reminder of the improvements made to assessment methods in medical education.

A third theme that runs through the book is that of technology. There are images of simulators, audio equipment and lantern screens. Many of the images demonstrate as much about our relationship with technology as they do about the technology itself. Technology has always been a part of medical education – however, it serves us best when it is the education that drives the technology rather than the other way around. Unfortunately, technology in medical education has not always worked like this. There are numerous examples where new technology promised to revolutionise medical curricula – only for the revolution to fizzle out a few years later. Film promised to transform medical education in the 1930s, television to do the same in the 1960s and then computers in the 1990s (7). A constant search for new innovations must always be balanced by a realistic evaluation of what they have achieved and what they can achieve.

There are a variety of different types of images in the book. One form of image that commonly features is the portrait. The purpose of a portrait is to show more than simply an exact representation of a person – the portrait typically suggests the person's personality or mood. This is true of portrait photography and painting. Portraits are typically posed and the subject usually looks directly at the camera or painter. The portraits in this book are no different, and many of them suggest common themes in medical education. The subjects in the portraits are serious or composed and wear formal or academic dress. Some have kindly expressions, but most are austere. What messages do these posed images convey about medical education and medical education leadership? I would argue that they suggest that medical education is a formal, solitary and serious business. However, this conception is diametrically opposite to what we know works best in medical education – that is activities that are informal, fun and carried out in groups.

Another common type of image is the caricature. The purpose of caricature is to amuse or to make a point or sometimes to do both. The point made may be complimentary of the subject but more commonly is critical and the criticism may be gently mocking or brutally wounding. The caricature is often less about the subject's appearance and more about their personality. Most of the caricatures in this book are of the gentle variety – however, they are no less insightful for that. Oliver Wendell Holmes, for example, is portrayed as an avuncular eccentric – academic yet approachable. These are all features that we would be happy to see in our modern medical teachers.

Some of the images are of statues. Why would some figures from the history of medical education be portrayed as statues? From prehistory, statues were created to commemorate a famous or influential person or a god. Did those who commissioned statues of figures from medical education intend to portray these figures as superhumans? It is certainly possible. However, another factor that shows the complexity of interpreting artefacts is that we tend to consider statues as stark and austere figures – the colour of hard stone. But recent research has shown that ancient statues were originally painted in bright colours. This in turn changes our perception of statues and also our perception as to how they were viewed in the past.

The images in this book show people portrayed as gods, deities, idols and sometimes supernatural beings. But the truth is that most of them were simply people – albeit people who were to have a profound effect on medicine. As we look to the future of medicine and medical education, we should remember them and build on their legacy.

References

1. de Bellaigue C. Introduction. In: Kapuscinski R, *Shah of Shahs*. Penguin Classics, London, 2006.

2. Frenk J, Chen L, Bhutta ZA, Cohen J, Crisp N, Evans T, Fineberg H et al. Health professionals for a new century: Transforming education to strengthen health systems in an interdependent world. *Lancet* 2010;376(9756):1923–1958.

3. Allbutt TC. An Address on medical education in London: Delivered at King's College Hospital on October 3rd, 1905, at the Opening of the Medical Session. *BMJ* 1905;2:913.

4. Copland J. The Hippocratic Oath. *The London Medical Repository* 1825;23(135):258. http://en.wikipedia.org/wiki/Hippocratic_Oath (accessed 1 May 2015).

5. Hippocrates. *The Law of Hippocrates*. 2004. http://www.gutenberg.org/cache/epub/5694/pg5694.html (accessed 1 May 2015).

6. Hull G. The influence of Herman Boerhaave. *J R Soc Med* 1997;90:512–514.

7. Walsh K. When innovation was young. *Med Educ* 2015;49(3):341–342.

Further Reading

Anderson J, Barnes E, Shackleton E. *The Art of Medicine: Over 2,000 Years of Images and Imagination*. University of Chicago Press: Chicago, IL, 2012.

Fox DM, Lawrence C. *Photographing Medicine: Images and Power in Britain and America since 1840*. Greenwood Press: New York, 1988.

Porter R. *The Cambridge Illustrated History of Medicine*. Cambridge University Press: Cambridge, UK, 2001.

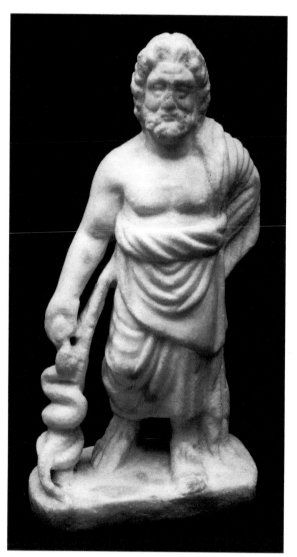

Asclepius was a Greco-Roman god who was associated with healing and medicine. It was believed that he cured the sick while they slept in a temple dedicated to him. This is known as incubation. In mythology, Asclepius was also said to be able to resurrect the dead. The statue shown in this figure was purchased in Istanbul, Turkey, in 1931. Maker: Unknown. (Credit: Science Museum, London, Wellcome Images [1].)

1 ASCLEPIUS

Asclepius was the Greek god of medicine and healing. He received instruction in medicine from the centaur Chiron. He cured the sick while they slept in a temple dedicated to him – this was known as incubation. He developed such expertise that he was able to bring people back from the dead. Some versions of the myth say that this caused overpopulation and so Asclepius was killed. Other versions say that he was killed for reviving Hippolytus and receiving gold as recompense. Other versions still say that Hades asked Zeus to kill him as he was worried that no more dead spirits would come to his underworld.

Asclepius had five daughters: Hygieia, the goddess of hygiene; Iaso, the goddess of recuperation; Aceso, the goddess of healing; Aglaea, the goddess of beauty; and Panacea, the goddess of universal cure. Emphasising the importance of Asclepius, the Hippocratic Oath began as follows: 'I swear by Apollo the Physician and by Asclepius and by Hygieia and Panacea and by all the gods…'.

This marble statue shows Asclepius as an old man – wise, strong and benign. The rod of Asclepius, a snake wrapped around a staff, is also visible – this remains the most common symbol of medicine to this day. The statue was purchased in Istanbul, Turkey, in 1931. Its maker is unknown.

Note

1. Copyrighted work available under Creative Commons Attribution only licence CC BY 4.0, http://creativecommons.org/licenses/by/4.0.

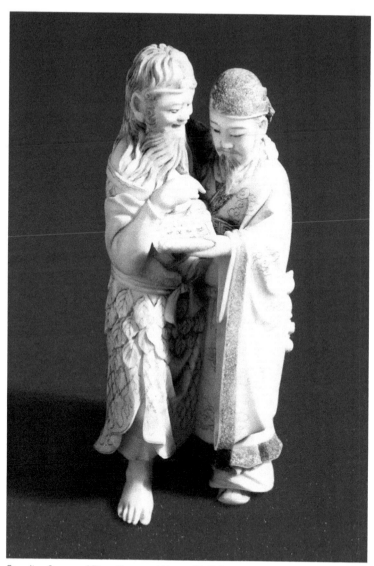

Standing figures of Shen Nung and Huang Ti, 7.5 cm. Carved Ivory.
(Credit: Wellcome Library [l].)

2 STANDING FIGURES OF SHEN NUNG AND HUANG TI

Shen Nung (third millennium BC) is considered the father of Chinese medicine. Huang Ti (also from the third millennium BC) co-authored *The Yellow Emperor's Canon of Internal Medicine* with Ch'i Po. This book is perhaps most interesting for its format: it consists of a series of questions posed by the Yellow Emperor and answered by the experts – a form of medical learning that continues to this day. George Brown (2) emphasises this: 'Questioning is one of the most widely used skills of medical teaching'. The answers to the Yellow Emperor's questions are long and detailed and give us a comprehensive view of what was known of medicine at the time. Interestingly some answers are more in keeping with the philosophy of the time in China than with what must have been known as anatomical fact – a tendency that finds resonance through the ages in medical education. Also of note is that physicians were advised to be mindful: they were instructed to time the patient's pulse according to their own respiratory rate and so had to be in good health before undertaking the consultation (the pulse was all important in diagnosis).

Here the ivory figures appear to be holding a scroll – perhaps it is the Canon itself.

Notes

1. Copyrighted work available under Creative Commons Attribution only licence CC BY 2.0, see http://creativecommons.org/licenses/by/2.0/.
2. Brown G. Self assessment. *Med Teach* 1983;5(1):27–29.

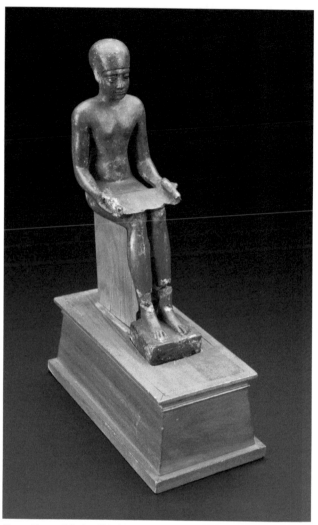

Place: Egypt. Made: 600–30 BCE. L0057137. (Credit: Science Museum, London, Wellcome Images [1].)

3 IMHOTEP

Imhotep (circa 2650–2600 BC) was an Egyptian physician, priest and god. He is often suggested as the author of the Edwin Smith Papyrus, which outlined detailed anatomical and pathological observations (Edwin Smith was the dealer who first bought it). The descriptions were based on case histories – Imhotep is the earliest advocate of this teaching method. Case-based learning is ubiquitous in healthcare professional education today.

And what exactly do we mean by case-based learning? The following is a useful description: 'basic, social and clinical sciences are studied in relation to the case, are integrated with clinical presentations and conditions (including health and ill-health) and student learning is, therefore, associated with real-life situations' (2). There is unquestionably good evidence that case-based learning is popular amongst learners. Tutors appear to enjoy this method also. Finally, case-based learning appears to promote self-directed learning and rational clinical problem-solving. Imhotep would likely have approved of this retrospective justification of his methods.

However, it wasn't all seriousness in Imhotep's teachings. The advice 'eat, drink and be merry for tomorrow we shall die' has been attributed to many sources – but perhaps the earliest attribution is to Imhotep (3).

Imhotep is typically shown in this pose – carefully studying a sheet of papyrus.

Notes

1. Copyrighted work available under Creative Commons Attribution only licence CC BY 4.0, http://creativecommons.org/licenses/by/4.0/.

2. Thistlethwaite JE, Davies D, Ekeocha S, Kidd JM, MacDougall C, Matthews P, Purkis J, Clay D. The effectiveness of case-based learning in health professional education. A BEME systematic review: BEME Guide No. 23. *Med Teach* 2012;34(6):e421–e444.

3. http://www.experienceproject.com/stories/Love-Inspirational-Quotes/618984 (accessed 10 March 2014).

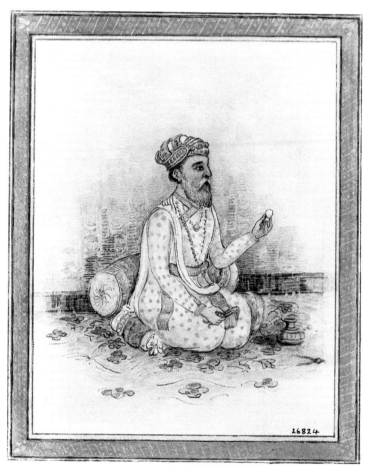

Watercolour drawing: portrait of Susruta. Watercolour by: H. Solomon.
(Credit: Wellcome Library [1].)

4 SUSRUTA

Susruta was an Indian physician, surgeon and author who probably lived in the sixth century BC. Little is known of his life. He was likely the author of the *Sushruta Samhita* – a comprehensive textbook on medicine and surgery. The *Sushruta Samhita* is remarkable for its ambition and range. It describes a variety of communicable and non-communicable diseases (including diabetes, obesity, heart disease, hypertension and leprosy). Perhaps most extraordinary is the text's section on plastic surgery: it mentions the use of flaps for a number of different purposes and also gives a basic outline on how to reconstruct the nose after an injury.

The text also touches on how best to study medicine: it suggests a programmatic approach and emphasises the importance of good study habits: 'A pupil who is pure, obedient to his preceptor, applies himself steadily to his work, and abandons laziness and excessive sleep, will arrive at the end of the science he has been studying' (2).

This watercolour depicts Susruta clearly, but what is he showing? Could it be a fruit or a stone in his left hand? In his right hand, he seems to be holding an instrument – its head is shaped like that of a bird.

Notes

1. Copyrighted work available under Creative Commons Attribution only licence CC BY 2.0, see http://creativecommons.org/licenses/by/2.0/.
2. *Sushruta Samhita*, 'Sutrasthanam', Ch. 1, see https://archive.org/stream/englishtranslati00susruoft/englishtranslati00susruoft_djvu.txt (accessed 8 March 2016).

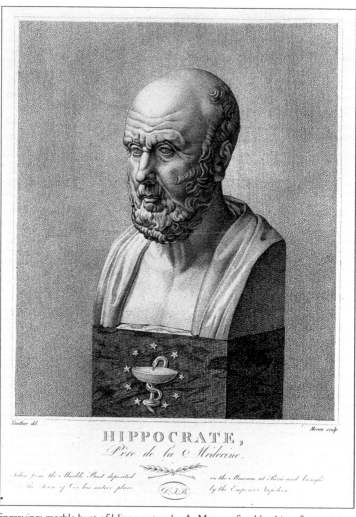

Engraving: marble bust of Hippocrates; by A. Mecou after Vauthier after a statue in the Louvre, n.d. Library reference no.: Burgess, Portraits, 1403.5. (Credit: Wellcome Library [1].)

5 HIPPOCRATES

Hippocrates (460–370 BC) was a Greek physician and classical scholar. He was born in Kos – but apart from that, little is known of his life. He is widely regarded as the father of medicine. He was the first to describe many diseases and also to set out standards of ethical behaviour to which physicians were expected to adhere. He realised the vast amount of learning required to practice medicine – impossible for a person to learn even in a lifetime: 'Life is short, the art long' (2). Many of Hippocrates' ideas and theories were subsequently proved to be wrong; however, he was the first to dispel the myth that diseases were punishments from the gods (he believed that they were caused by natural phenomena). He was the first to describe many signs and diseases – from clubbing to empyema. He classified diseases as acute or chronic and described the natural history of many diseases – from onset to convalescence.

Hippocrates was first and foremost a kind physician. He advised rest, balms, hygiene and occasional medications. The purpose of medicine was to help nature apply its natural healing powers and to avoid doing harm.

This bust is a typical portrayal of Hippocrates – as an experienced and wise old man.

Notes

1. Copyrighted work available under Creative Commons Attribution only licence CC BY 2.0, see http://creativecommons.org/licenses/by/2.0/.
2. http ://www.brainyquote.com/quotes/authors/h/hippocrates.html (accessed 10 March 2014).

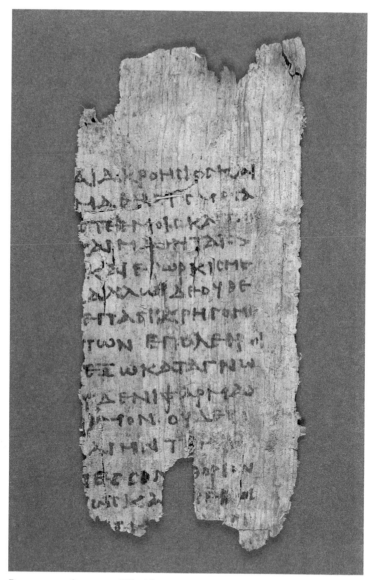

Papyrus text: fragment of The Hippocratic Oath: verso, showing oath.
Library reference no.: External Reference Oxyrhynchus papyri no. 2547.
(Credit: Wellcome Library [1].)

6 PAPYRUS TEXT: FRAGMENT OF THE HIPPOCRATIC OATH

The Hippocratic Oath is taken by physicians who promise to practice medicine to high ethical and professional standards. Physicians who take the oath also promise to respect those who have taught them medicine and to pass medical education on to the sons of their instructors, to their own sons and to others who have taken the oath. The oath also emphasises the importance of safe practice: 'I will prescribe regimens for the good of my patients according to my ability and my judgment and never do harm to anyone'. In taking the oath, physicians promise not to encroach onto the specialist domains of other practitioners such as surgeons. Physicians also promise to maintain confidentiality and not to mislead patients or take advantage of them. Ironically although the oath is inextricably linked to his name, it is not certain that Hippocrates actually wrote it. It may have originated after his death.

The oath is rarely taken today but has inspired other attempts to define good practice. For example, the General Medical Council issues guidance on good medical practice for doctors working in the United Kingdom.

This torn papyrus text shows a fragment of the oath.

Note

1. Copyrighted work available under Creative Commons Attribution only licence CC BY 2.0, see http://creativecommons.org/licenses/by/2.0.

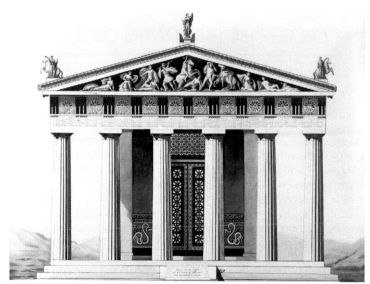

Reconstruction of the facade of the temple of Asclepius at Epidaurus. Watercolour. From: Epidaure, restauration & description des principaux monuments du sanctuaire d'Asclépios. By: Defrasse, Alphonse and Lechat, Henri. Published: Librairies-Imprimeries Reunies Paris 1895. Plate III. (Credit: Wellcome Library [1].)

7 FACADE OF THE TEMPLE OF ASCLEPIUS AT EPIDAURUS

The temple of Asclepius at Epidaurus was built in the fourth century BC. Asclepius was the Greek god of medicine and healing. Only the foundation of the temple is preserved. Medicine and medical education have had an association with religion for centuries. According to Kenneth Hill, 'historically the training of medical men from the earliest times has had a cultural association, particularly with religion. Thus the witch-doctor (with his psychosomatic associations) and the priests of ancient times (with access to the gods of health) tended to underline the importance of medicine as an art or mystique rather than the application of pure techniques' (2). The first treatments for diseases were often religious prayers, dances or ceremonies. Religious shamans used magical cures. Over the millennia, medicine has developed as a science and has slowly shed its religious origins. However, many remnants remain. Latin continues to have a strong influence over the language of both religion and medicine. The title 'dean' may describe someone who holds a position of authority in the church or in medical education.

This image shows a reconstruction. However, the original temple was to have a long-lasting influence on the architecture of buildings associated with medical education. This influence can be seen in other images in this book – such as that showing the buildings in Harvard's 'Great White Quadrangle' (Image 98) and the School of Surgery in Paris (Image 49).

Notes

1. Copyrighted work available under Creative Commons Attribution only licence CC BY 4.0, http://creativecommons.org/licenses/by/4.0/.
2. Hill KR. Some reflections on medical education and teaching in the developing countries. *BMJ* 1962;2:585.

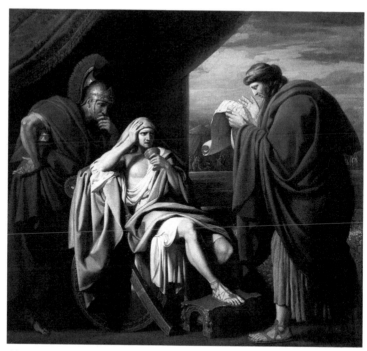

Alexander the Great's confidence in his physician Philip of Acarnania. Oil painting by Benjamin West. (Credit: Wellcome Library [1].)

8 ALEXANDER THE GREAT'S CONFIDENCE IN HIS PHYSICIAN PHILIP OF ACARNANIA

Philip of Acarnania was the physician of Alexander the Great. In 333 BC, Alexander had been warned of being assassinated by poisoning; however, he readily drank the medicine for fever prepared for him by Philip. Alexander made a quick and full recovery. In the scene, Alexander is about to drink and yet keeps his eyes focussed on Philip. The painting is by Benjamin West, an American painter of historical scenes.

It is uncertain whether Philip was present some years later when Alexander claimed 'I am dying with the help of too many physicians'. These famous last words seem to encapsulate the problem of patients who have seen too many physicians and yet have not got any better. Communication between physician and physician, between physician and interdisciplinary team members, and between physician and patient is key to solving this dilemma. Communication skills teaching has become part of modern medical education curricula and yet the problem remains. Recent thinking is that communication skills training should not be separated from the rest of the curriculum, but rather it should be an integral part of all components. Students should thus learn to integrate communication and clinical skills and to practice both skills in context.

However, the communication skills of Philip in this picture are questionable. He is reading a scroll and studiously avoids eye contact with his patient.

Note

1. Copyrighted work available under Creative Commons Attribution only licence CC BY 2.0, see http://creativecommons.org/licenses/by/2.0.

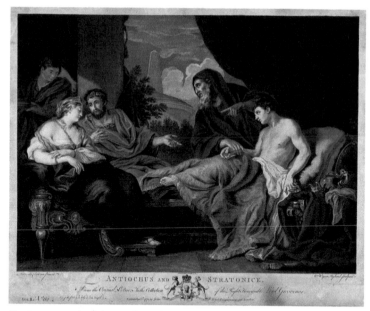

Erasistratus, a physician, realising that Antiochus's (son of Seleucus I) illness is lovesickness for his stepmother Stratonice, by observing that Antiochus's pulse rose whenever he saw her. Coloured engraving by W.W. Ryland, 1772, after Pietro da Cortona. 1772. Published: John Boydell, London (engraver in Cheapside): 1 September 1772. (Credit: Wellcome Library [1].)

9 ERASISTRATUS, A PHYSICIAN, REALISING THAT ANTIOCHUS'S ILLNESS IS LOVESICKNESS FOR HIS STEPMOTHER STRATONICE, BY OBSERVING THAT ANTIOCHUS'S PULSE ROSE WHENEVER HE SAW HER

Erasistratus (304–250 BC) was a Greek physician and anatomist. He founded a medical school in Alexandria. He was the first to describe the valves of the heart and to realise that the heart was a pump. He was also interested in learning. According to Erasistratus, 'people who are unused to learning learn little, and that slowly, while those more accustomed do much more and do it more easily' (2).

In modern medical schools, this concept might be translated as learning to learn. At a time when train the trainers courses in medical education are flourishing, there is an argument for having complementary learning to learn courses. Certainly some students enter medical school with poor learning skills. Often the skills that have gotten them into medical school will no longer be capable of helping them navigate a complicated curriculum with multiple components. Learning by rote will no longer be enough. Students must learn the skills of interpreting data, integrating knowledge and applying sometimes academic ideas to the real world.

In this image, Erasistratus shows the benefits of lifelong learning. He is unlikely to have seen a case like this before but quickly realises that Antiochus's illness is lovesickness for his stepmother Stratonice. He comes to this conclusion by observing that Antiochus's pulse rose whenever he saw her. Erasistratus not only diagnoses the illness, he also provides a cure – he convinces Antiochus's father (Seleucus I) to give up his wife for his son.

Notes

1. Copyrighted work available under Creative Commons Attribution only licence CC BY 2.0, see http://creativecommons.org/licenses/by/2.0/.

2. 'On paralysis'. Quoted in A. J. Brock, *Greek Medicine: Being Extracts Illustrative of Medical Writers from Hippocrates to Galen*, 1929, p. 185.

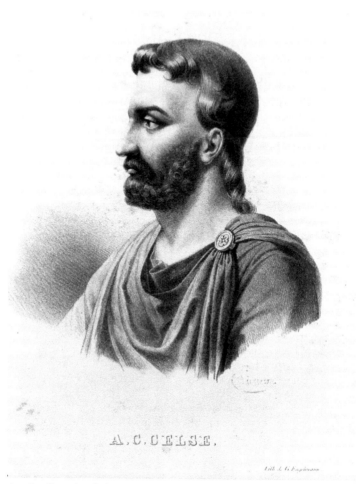

A. C. CELSE.

Aurelius Cornelius Celsus. Lithograph by P. R. Vigneron. Lithograph 1820/1829. (Credit: Wellcome Library [1].)

10 CELSUS

Aulus Cornelius Celsus (circa 25 BC–circa 50 AD) was a Roman writer and encyclopaedist. His great work was *De Medicina* which described medicine, pharmacy and surgery in the Roman world. He may not actually have been a practicing physician at all but rather a writer on a range of topics from medicine to military matters. He made major contributions to the specialty of dermatology – the disease kerion celsi still bears his name. Celsus was the first to describe something which every medical student would still recognise – the features of inflammation. In Celsus's terms these were rubor, calor, dolor and tumor (redness, heat, pain and swelling respectively). The fifth feature 'loss of function' was added later.

Celsus wrote about best practice in communicating with patients and about the skills required of a competent surgeon. Little is known of his life apart from that which can be gleaned from the content of his medical writings and his elegant Latin prose style. His most famous quote was 'live in rooms full of light' – this is likely to be advice to patients but perhaps it is not too fanciful to suggest that he may have been referring to enlightenment in medical thinking and learning (2).

Notes

1. Copyrighted work available under Creative Commons Attribution only licence CC BY 2.0, see http://creativecommons.org/licenses/by/2.0/.
2. http://izquotes.com/author/a.-cornelius-celsus (accessed 9 March 2016).

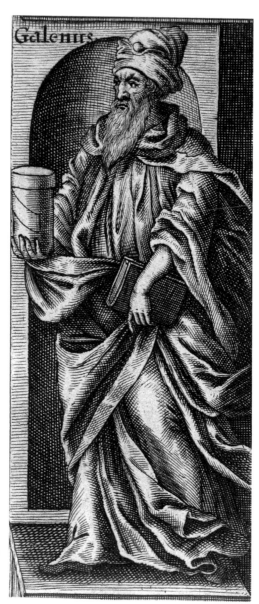

GALEN {c. 130–200}. Line engraving: portrait of Galen holding book and ointment jar; anon., n.d. {seventeenth century}. Library reference no.: Burgess, Portraits 1069.7. (Credit: Wellcome Library [1].)

11 GALEN

Galen (129–200) was a Roman researcher, surgeon, philosopher and anatomist. He felt that medical knowledge was made up of logic, physics and ethics and that physicians needed an education in all three. He was surgeon to the gladiators and thus perfected his knowledge of wound management. However, his knowledge of anatomy was based not on human dissection but on the dissection of monkeys and pigs (this is because Rome had banned the dissection of human cadavers).

Galen's ideas were to influence Western medical science for more than 1000 years. Many of his ideas were correct – for example, he discovered that the voice comes from the larynx. However, many were incorrect and were to mislead physicians for centuries – for example, his belief that venous blood was created in the liver and arterial blood in the heart.

Galen was a strong advocate of ongoing learning and keeping an open mind: 'The fact is that those who are enslaved to their sects are not merely devoid of all sound knowledge, but they will not even stop to learn!' (2)

This line engraving shows Galen in action – sallying forth holding a book and an ointment jar.

Notes

1. Copyrighted work available under Creative Commons Attribution only licence CC BY 2.0, see http://creativecommons.org/licenses/by/2.0.
2. *On the Natural Faculties*, Bk. 1, sect. 13; cited from Arthur John Brock (trans.), *On the Natural Faculties*. London, UK: Heinemann; 1963, p. 57.

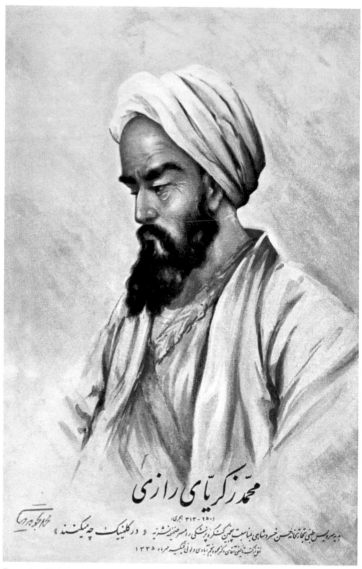

Portrait of Rhazes (al-Razi) (AD 865–925) physician and alchemist who lived in Baghdad. (Credit: Wellcome Library [I].)

12 RHAZES

Rhazes (AD 865–925) was born Muhammad ibn Zakariyā Rāzī in Rey, Persia. He was a physician, philosopher and chemist. He was also a prolific author – writing more than 200 manuscripts in his lifetime. He wrote about infectious diseases (including smallpox and measles), and his ideas were to have influence throughout the world for many centuries.

His medical teaching was often based on the questions of his students; however, he always allowed other students to attempt to answer questions before he intervened. This method of peer education persists to this day. He also wrote about the ethics of medicine: 'the doctor's aim is to do good, even to our enemies, so much more to our friends, and my profession forbids us to do harm to our kindred, as it is instituted for the benefit and welfare of the human race, and God imposed on physicians the oath not to compose mortiferous remedies' (2).

According to the science historian George Sartan, 'Rhazes was the greatest physician of Islam and the Medieval Ages' (3). The Razi Institute in Tehran is named after him and an annual 'Razi Day' ('Pharmacy Day') is still held in his honour in Iran.

Notes

1. Copyrighted work available under Creative Commons Attribution only licence CC BY 2.0, see http://creativecommons.org/licenses/by/2.0/.

2. *Islamic Science, the Scholar and Ethics*, Foundation for Science Technology and Civilisation, see http://www.muslimheritage.com/article/islamic-science-scholar-and-ethics (accessed 9 March 2016).

3. Sarton G. *Introduction to the History of Science*, Vol. 1. Baltimore, MD: Williams and Wilkins; 1927–1948, p. 609.

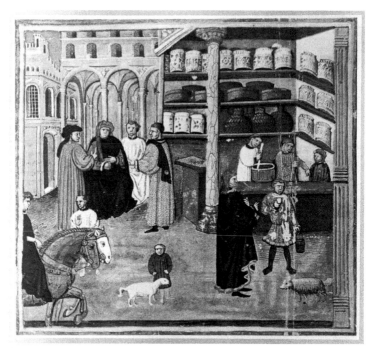

Avicenna expounding pharmacy to his pupils, from the fifteenth century "Great Cannon of Avicenna" From: Sixty Centuries of Health and Physick. (Credit: Wellcome Library [1].)

13 AVICENNA EXPOUNDING PHARMACY TO HIS PUPILS

Avicenna (980–1037) was a Persian philosopher, astronomer and physician. He wrote two books – *The Book of Healing* and *The Canon of Medicine* – both of which became standard medical textbooks in medical schools throughout the Middle Ages. He was interested in medical knowledge and learning in their widest senses: 'Now it is established in the sciences that no knowledge is acquired save through the study of its causes and beginnings, if it has had causes and beginnings; nor completed except by knowledge of its accidents and accompanying essentials' (2). Aetiology and pathophysiology remain core components of medical curricula to this day. The Canon is prescient in its description of how to test medicines. Avicenna advises that medicines should be tested on simple diseases; that they should be tested on more than one disease; that they should be tested so that their actions are consistent and timely; and that they should be tested on humans.

Here is Avicenna expounding pharmacy to his students: the scene is striking for the activity in the learning environment. Learners are gesticulating, stirring, carrying out tasks.

Notes

1. Copyrighted work available under Creative Commons Attribution only licence CC BY 2.0, see http://creativecommons.org/licenses/by/2.0/.
2. http://www.brainyquote.com/quotes/authors/a/avicenna.html (accessed 10 March 2014).

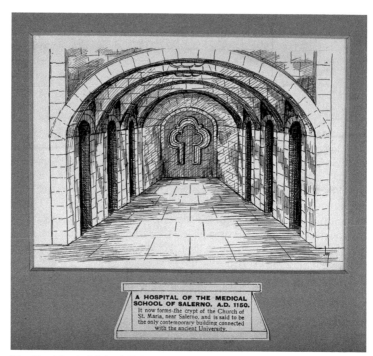

A HOSPITAL OF THE MEDICAL
SCHOOL OF SALERNO, A.D. 1150.
It now forms the crypt of the Church of
St. Maria, near Salerno, and is said to be
the only contemporary building connected
with the ancient University.

Teaching Hospital School, Salerno, Italy: part of the Crypt of St Maria. Pen and ink drawing. (Credit: Wellcome Library [1].)

14 TEACHING HOSPITAL SCHOOL, SALERNO, ITALY

The medical school at Salerno was founded in 1096. It was the first European school to develop the core aspects of medical education that we still recognise today – a curriculum, a formal assessment and a form of internship.

The school produced one of the earliest textbooks of medicine, *Regimen Sanitatis Salernitanum*, which contained much useful advice about the practice of medicine. 'Use three physicians still; first Doctor Quiet next Doctor Merryman and Doctor Dyet' (2). The textbook covers many ancient treatments and also gives important advice about professional conduct:

Good common sense and leechcraft cure disease,
Not empty words of boastful, lying quack;
The first combined give suff'ring mortals ease,
The last to perish, leave them on the rack.

It also touches on the limitations of medicine:

Were doctors skilled enough to undermine
Each fell disease, they'd almost be divine.
But, as all practice shows, no doctor can
Make life anew, though he may stretch its span.

This drawing shows part of the Crypt of the Church of St Maria. It is the only remaining part of the original university.

Notes

1. Copyrighted work available under Creative Commons Attribution only licence CC BY 2.0, see http://creativecommons.org/licenses/by/2.0/.
2. *Regimen Sanitatis Salernitanum*. Translated by J. Harrington. Salerno, Campania: Ente Provinciale per il Turismo; 1966, p. 22.

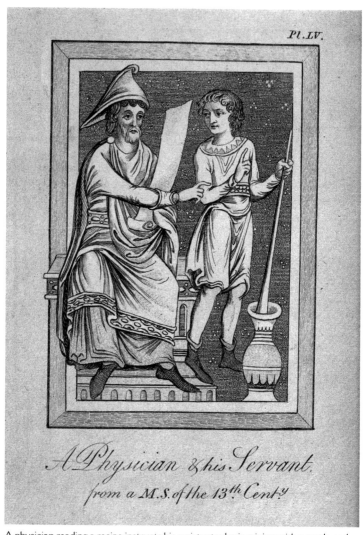

A physician reading a recipe instructs his assistant who is mixing with a pestle and mortar. Engraving after a twelfth century manuscript. (Credit: Wellcome Library [1].)

15 A PHYSICIAN READING A RECIPE INSTRUCTS HIS ASSISTANT

There has always been a tension between training and education in medical schools. Training typically involves instruction on how to carry out a skill, whereas education involves drawing out knowledge, skills and behaviours from the learner. Training is about developing competencies in various activities; however, education is about developing professionals and engendering lifelong learning and decision-making skills so that learners know when to apply what they have learned. Ultimately education creates independent thinkers, whereas training produces people who are able to carry out set tasks. It is not that one is better than the other – they both have an important role to play. Sometimes both will be used in the same course. According to Willoughby Francis Wade, 'it is, I suppose, impossible to instruct a person without in some degree educating him, or to educate without in some degree instructing him' (2).

This engraving suggests gentle instruction. The physician is reading a recipe to his assistant who in turn is mixing the treatment with a pestle and mortar. Both figures know their role, they are carrying out their tasks, and they seem to have a rapport. The trainer (or educator) is certainly close at hand and available to the learner.

Notes

1. Copyrighted work available under Creative Commons Attribution only licence CC BY 4.0, http://creativecommons.org/licenses/by/4.0/.
2. Wade WF. President's address, delivered at the fifty-eighth annual meeting of the British Medical Association. *BMJ* 1890;2:259.

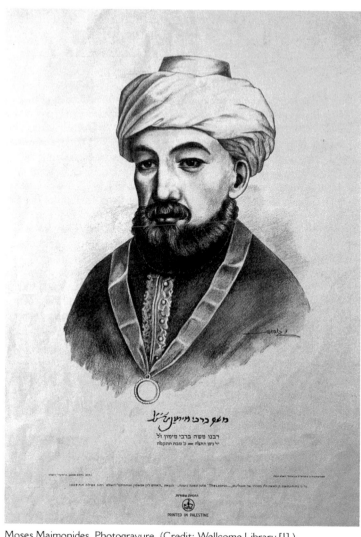

Moses Maimonides. Photogravure. (Credit: Wellcome Library [I].)

16 MAIMONIDES

Moses Maimonides (1135–1204) was a scholar and physician from the Middle Ages. He studied medicine in Córdoba and Fes and was eventually appointed physician to the Grand Vizier and then to the Sultan Saladin. He published extensively on medical matters. His noted works include *Commentary on the Aphorisms of Hippocrates, Medical Aphorisms of Moses, Regimen of Health* and *Glossary of Drug Names*. He described many communicable and non-communicable diseases (from hepatitis to diabetes).

Maimonides was dedicated to his craft – after a day in court he would typically arrive home to more people waiting for him: 'Jews and Mohammedans, prominent and unimportant, friends and enemies, a varied crowd, who are looking for my medical advice. There is scarcely time for me to get down from my carriage and wash myself and eat a little, and then until night I am constantly occupied, so that, from sheer exhaustion, I must lie down. Only on the Sabbath day have I the time to occupy myself with my own people and my studies, and so the day is away from me' (2).

Despite his many achievements, he remained a humble man and lifelong scholar: 'Grant me an opportunity to improve and extend my training, since there is no limit to knowledge' (3).

Maimonides had one son who survived into adulthood, Avraham. He in turn became a scholar and physician as did subsequent generations of the family.

Notes

1. Copyrighted work available under Creative Commons Attribution only licence CC BY 2.0, see http://creativecommons.org/licenses/by/2.0/.
2. http://www.gutenberg.org/files/20216/20216-h/20216-h.htm#Page_90 (accessed 15 April 2015).
3. Mishneh Torah, Ch. IV, p. 19.

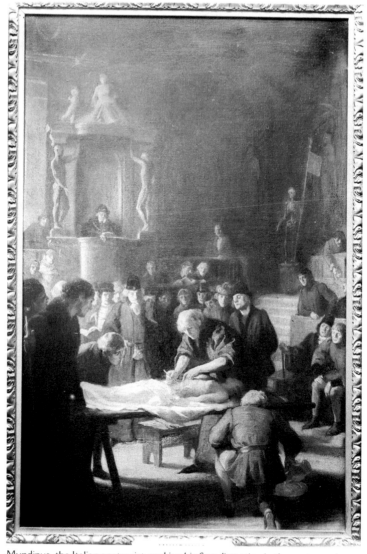

Mundinus, the Italian anatomist, making his first dissection in the anatomy theatre at Bologna, 1318. Oil painting by Ernest Board. Circa 1910. (Credit: Wellcome Library [1].)

17 MUNDINUS, THE ITALIAN ANATOMIST, MAKING HIS FIRST DISSECTION

Mundinus (circa 1270–1326) was born Mondino de Luzzi in Bologna, Italy. He was an anatomist, surgeon and teacher. Unconventionally for the time, Mundinus performed anatomical dissections himself (rather than use a demonstrator). He is often called the 'restorer of anatomy' as he reintroduced the practice of anatomical dissections into medical curricula (2).

Mundinus was also an author – his great work was *Anathomia corporis humani*. It was widely used throughout Europe for 300 years after its first publication. *Anathomia corporis humani* is based on Mundinus' own experiences in conducting dissections and also on the writings of the ancient scholars (such as Hippocrates and Galen). Some of the errors of these predecessors were repeated in Mundinus' own text. This tendency to continue to follow the guidance of earlier scholars is as old as science itself. It is certainly worthwhile taking older writings into account but occasionally new beliefs must be followed. According to Jennifer Leaning, 'Hippocrates and Maimonides still abide, but the vast changes in situation and circumstance since they spoke create the need for other canons' (3).

This image catches the excitement of the learners at this first dissection. One leans forward; another peers over the shoulder of the dissector; others are more hesitant and look on from what they might feel is a safe distance. The picture is by Ernest Board, an English painter who specialised in historical and mythical subjects, and portraits.

Notes

1. Copyrighted work available under Creative Commons Attribution only licence CC BY 2.0, see http://creativecommons.org/licenses/by/2.0/.
2. http://en.wikipedia.org/wiki/Mondino_de_Liuzzi#CITEREFSinger1957 (accessed 18 March 2016).
3. Leaning J. Human rights and medical education: Why every medical student should learn the Universal Declaration of Human Rights. *BMJ* 1997;315:1390.

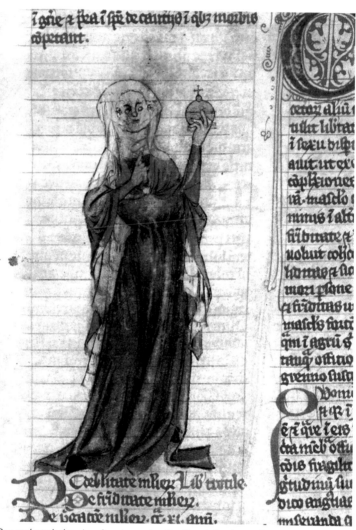

Pen and wash drawing showing a standing female healer, perhaps of Trotula, clothed in red and green with a white headdress, holding up a urine flask to which she points with her right hand. Early fourteenth century. From: Miscellanea medica XVIII. Folio 65 recto (=33 recto). (Credit: Wellcome Library [l].)

18 TROTULA

Trotula was an Italian gynaecologist and educator at the medical school in Salerno. She wrote books on women's health – her goal was to help male doctors learn about the female body. Little is known about the life of Trotula – indeed there is controversy as to whether she actually existed. Nonetheless the books are thought to be the 'most popular assembly of materials on women's medicine from the late twelfth through the fifteenth centuries' (2). The titles of the books are *Book on the Conditions of Women*, *On Treatments for Women* and *On Women's Cosmetics*. *Book on the Conditions of Women* covers topics such as pregnancy and childbirth, menstruation and the care of the newborn child. *On Treatments for Women* emphasises treatments to ensure fertility – clearly an important topic at the time. The text explains what medications to give but gives no rationale as to how or why they work. The final text *On Women's Cosmetics* deals with how best to use cosmetics to enhance female beauty.

This pen and wash drawing shows a female figure 'perhaps of Trotula, clothed in red and green with a white headdress, holding up a urine flask to which she points with her right hand' (3).

Notes

1. Copyrighted work available under Creative Commons Attribution only licence CC BY 2.0, see http://creativecommons.org/licenses/by/2.0/.

2. Green MH, *Women's Healthcare in the Medieval West: Texts and Contexts*. Aldershot, UK: Ashgate; 2000, Appendix, pp. 1–36.

3. http://wellcomeimages.org/.

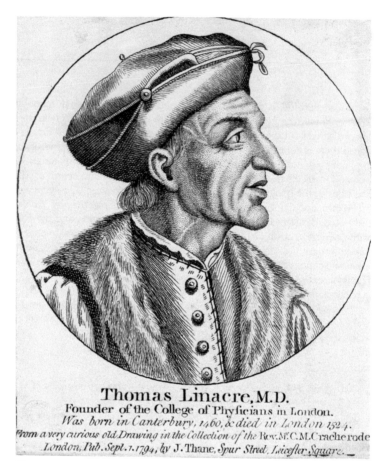

Thomas Linacre. Engraving, 1794. (Credit: Wellcome Library [1].)

19 THOMAS LINACRE

Thomas Linacre (1460–1524) was an English physician and scholar. He translated many of the works of the ancient Greek physicians, thereby making them accessible to a wide audience. He studied in Italy and then returned to England eager to spread learning that was flowering at the time of the Italian Renaissance. Respected as much as a scholar as a physician, he was appointed tutor to Arthur – Prince of Wales – the older brother of Henry VIII. He was subsequently appointed physician to Henry VIII, Cardinal Wolsey and other Tudor luminaries.

Linacre founded the Royal College of Physicians of London and became its first president. According to the Roll of the College, 'the most magnificent of Linacre's labors was the design of the Royal College of Physicians of London – a standing monument of the enlightened views and generosity of its projectors. In the execution of it Linacre stood alone, for the munificence of the Crown was limited to a grant of letters patent; whilst the expenses and provision of the College was left to be defrayed out of his own means, or of those who were associated with him in its foundation' (2). Linacre left his house and library to the college when he died. It was then located in Knightrider Street in the City of London. Today the college 'occupies a tiny Vatican in Regents Park, whose benign soft-footed cardinals pad around discussing preferment of one kind or another' (3).

Notes

1. Copyrighted work available under Creative Commons Attribution only licence CC BY 2.0, see http://creativecommons.org/licenses/by/2.0/.
2. http://www.gutenberg.org/files/34067/34067-h/34067-h.htm#79 (accessed 19 April 2015).
3. Richards P, Stockill S, Foster R, Ingall E. *Learning Medicine*, 17th edn. Cambridge, UK: Cambridge University Press, 2006.

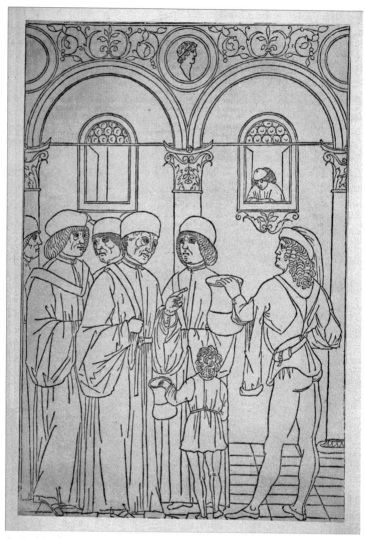

A physician lecturing to students about urinoscopy; he points to a flask held by an assistant. Heliotype. (Credit: Wellcome Library [1].)

20 A PHYSICIAN LECTURING TO STUDENTS ABOUT URINOSCOPY POINTS TO A FLASK HELD BY AN ASSISTANT

According to Swale Vincent, 'The formal lecture without demonstrations is a pitiable anachronism. It is a survival from the days when there were no textbooks' (2). The physician in this image was lecturing several hundred years before Vincent, and yet shows his understanding of the importance of demonstrations.

In the modern era, learning by means of demonstrations is just as important as ever. However, it is no longer good enough to follow the anachronistic approach of 'see one, do one, teach one'. Medical education has since moved on to the concept of Miller's pyramid of competence where learners climb the pyramid from 'knowing' to 'knowing how' to 'showing how' and finally to 'doing'. Even more recently, the educational model of entrustable professional activities has come to the fore. Entrustable professional activities 'are units of professional practice, defined as tasks or responsibilities to be entrusted to the unsupervised execution by a trainee once he or she has attained sufficient specific competence' (3). This paradigm allows medical teachers and their learners to make reliable decisions on the level of supervision that learners need when carrying out specific tasks. Entrustable professional activities are task or work dependent and they typically require the learner to put together a number of different competencies in carrying out the task. As such they are closer to the real world of clinical practice – as it is this ability to integrate skills and competencies that makes a good physician.

Notes

1. Copyrighted work available under Creative Commons Attribution only licence CC BY 2.0, see http://creativecommons.org/licenses/by/2.0.

2. Vincent S. Medical research and education. *BMJ* 1920;2:562.

3. ten Cate O. Nuts and bolts of entrustable professional activities. *J Grad Med Educ* 2013;5(1):157–158.

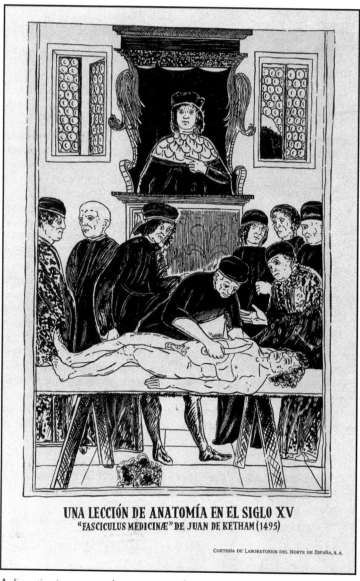

UNA LECCIÓN DE ANATOMÍA EN EL SIGLO XV
"FASCICULUS MEDICINÆ" DE JUAN DE KETHAM (1495)

CORTESÍA DE LABORATORIOS DEL NORTE DE ESPAÑA, S. A.

A dissection in progress: the anatomy professor at his lectern. Line block after a drawing after a woodcut, 1493. After: Mondino dei Luzzi. Published: Laboratorios del Norte de España [Spain]. (Credit: Wellcome Library [1].)

21 A DISSECTION IN PROGRESS: THE ANATOMY PROFESSOR AT HIS LECTERN

According to Henry Morris, 'dissection is the only perfect way of learning anatomy, which has been even defined as a "doctrine learned by dissections"' (2). This image shows the classic way of teaching and learning dissection. The professor is professing at his pulpit while the demonstrator performs the actual dissection. The students are merely observers. Reforms would lead to professors descending from their pulpits and doing the dissection and finally to the students themselves doing the dissections under supervision.

Today a variety of other means are used to teach anatomy. Learners may be provided with pre-dissected material. This gives more time for teaching and can be helpful if cadavers are scarce (because of a lack of donors). An alternative is to use life models – this method allows learners 'to see structures move and function' (3). A further alternative is to use radiological imaging techniques. Ultrasonography, computer-aided tomography, magnetic resonance imaging and positron emission tomography have all been used to teach anatomy. These modalities can demonstrate two- and three-dimensional still images of anatomical structures and organs or can show live movement (e.g. echocardiography). All these different methods have their place and it is unlikely that any one method is significantly better than the other. Decisions on whether to use particular methods should be based on the intended learning outcomes and what is available.

Notes

1. Copyrighted work available under Creative Commons Attribution only licence CC BY 4.0, http://creativecommons.org/licenses/by/4.0.
2. Morris H. A lecture introductory to the course on anatomy. *BMJ* 1876;2:515.
3. Collins J. Modern approaches to teaching and learning anatomy. *BMJ* 2008;337:a1310.

Surgeon with two students (or relatives of the patient?) by the bedside of a patient with a chest wound. Woodcut circa 1497. From: Das Buch der Cirurgia des Hieronymus Brunschwig. By: Hieronymus Brunschwig. Published: Druck und Verlag Carl Kuhn, München: 1911. (Credit: Wellcome Library [1].)

22 SURGEON WITH TWO STUDENTS (OR RELATIVES OF THE PATIENT) BY THE BEDSIDE OF A PATIENT WITH A CHEST WOUND

According to Thomas Lewis, 'The most fitted to teach practical medicine and surgery are those successfully and daily engaged in its practice' (2). Learning at the bedside has always been the cornerstone of medical and surgical education and certainly these students (if they are students) have a perfect view of the wound and any proceedings. The pose of the surgeon-educator is fascinating. Why is he holding up both hands? Is he calming the patient in distress or reassuring the students who also seem distressed?

Transitions in medical education are important and perhaps the most important transition is that from pre-clinical to clinical activities. Transitions are often times of stress and yet also great learning opportunities. Much recent research in medical education has concentrated on transitions. Modern thinking is that transitions should no longer be considered as inherently problematic but rather as ripe opportunities for learning from the new. Could this image show these students' first visit to the surgical ward? And could the surgeon-educator have managed the visit better? The image is from *Das Buch der Cirurgia* (*The Book of Surgery*) by Hieronymus Brunschwig (ca. 1450–ca. 1512).

Notes

1. Copyrighted work available under Creative Commons Attribution only licence CC BY 2.0, see http://creativecommons.org/licenses/by/2.

2. Lewis T. The Huxley lecture on clinical science within the university. *BMJ* 1935;1:631.

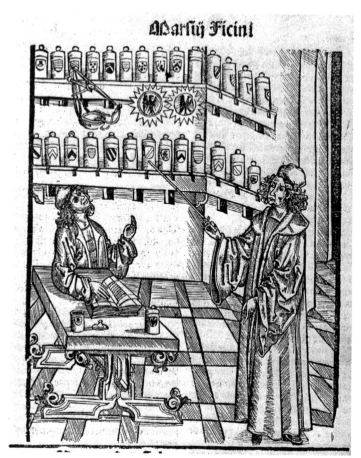

Pharmacy: master pointing at flasks and apprentice seated behind a desk. Woodcut. From: Medicinarius. Das Buch der Gesuntheit. By: Ficinus and Brunschwig. Published: J. Gruninger Strassburg 1505. Folio CXLII verso. (Credit: Wellcome Library [1].)

23 PHARMACY: MASTER POINTING AT FLASKS AND APPRENTICE SEATED BEHIND A DESK

The apprenticeship model of medical education has had its supporters and critics down through the ages. However, the debate about apprenticeship might be more fruitful if it concentrated less on its rights and wrongs and more on how the idea is actually implemented. Broadly, a successful apprenticeship means that the learner is actively involved in the task – this might mean assisting in a surgical procedure. The learner must also become socialised with the team and must interact with them and become part of their group. Thus, the age old model of apprenticeship in medical learning starts to sound remarkably like modern concepts such as 'legitimate peripheral participation' within 'communities of practice'.

Apprenticeships are not easy to set up within the modern clinical environment: clinicians are busier than ever before, patients can refuse to see medical students and attachments have become shorter. However, these obstacles can and must be overcome to ensure the delivery of relevant medical education to students. Here is David Wilson on how best to implement the apprenticeship model in medicine: 'surely the secret of a good apprenticeship is to have a good master, and the basic requirement for being a good master is to work alongside one's apprentices' (2).

Certainly master and apprentice are working side by side in this image. The learning is active: the figures are reading, demonstrating, maybe even asking and answering questions.

Notes

1. Copyrighted work available under Creative Commons Attribution only licence CC BY 4.0, http://creativecommons.org/licenses/by/4.0/.
2. Wilson DH. Teaching in casualty. *BMJ* 1982;285:1355.

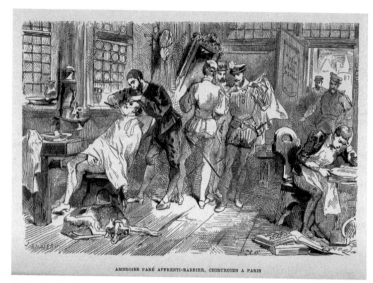

AMBROISE PARÉ APPRENTI-BARBIER, CHIRURGIEN A PARIS

Ambroise Paré, as an apprentice barber surgeon in a busy shop in Paris. Wood engraving by E. Morin after J. Ansseau. (Credit: Wellcome Library [1].)

24 AMBROISE PARÉ, AS AN APPRENTICE BARBER-SURGEON IN A BUSY SHOP IN PARIS

Ambroise Paré (1510–1590) was a French anatomist, military barber-surgeon and inventor of surgical instruments. He was an early promoter of the scientific method – often comparing wound treatments on different groups of patients. Even though clearly a talented surgeon and innovator, he remained modest about his achievements: 'I dressed him, and God healed him' (2). Paré wrote a fascinating account of his life as a military surgeon in *Journeys in Diverse Places*. In the text he writes, 'see how I learned to treat gunshot wounds; not by books' and gives detailed case histories of injured soldiers whom he treated (3). Paré is clearly learning by experience and is not just learning surgical methods: he is learning about how to work with colleagues and how to gain the trust of his patients. Like all authors, he was keen to pass on his experience to others.

The picture shows Paré at work – in a barber shop. Barber-surgeons were usually tasked with looking after wounded soldiers after a battle. They treated wounds, amputated limbs and sometimes even cut hair. Barber-surgeons were not physicians, and signs of their legacy exist to this day. The red and white barber's pole represents the blood and bandages applied by barber-surgeons to their patients. And surgeons in Britain are still called 'Mr' rather than 'Dr', as barber-surgeons did not have a university education.

Notes

1. Copyrighted work available under Creative Commons Attribution only licence CC BY 2.0, see http://creativecommons.org/licenses/by/2.0/.
2. Quoted in Francis Randolph Packard, 'The Voyages Made Into Divers Places: The Journey to Turin in 1536', *Life and Times of Ambroise Paré* 1510–1590.
3. http://www.gutenberg.org/cache/epub/5694/pg5694.html (accessed 18 April 2015).

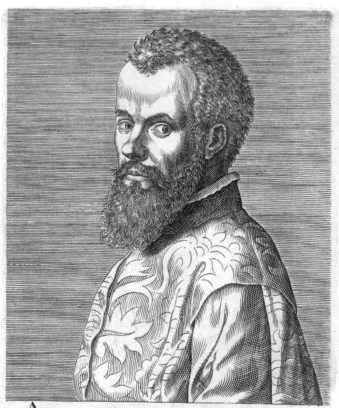

Portrait of Andreas Vesalius Bruxellensis Anatomicorum Facile Princeps. 1572.
From: Virorum doctorum de disciplinis bene merentium effigies XLIIII. Published:
P. Galle, Antuerpiae: 1572. (Credit: Wellcome Library [1].)

25 VESALIUS

Andreas Vesalius (1514–1564) was a Belgian physician and anatomist. He was professor of surgery at Padua – one of the leading medical schools of the day. He wrote *De Humani Corporis Fabrica*, which was to become an iconic textbook of anatomy. At the start of the sixteenth century, the works of Galen and other ancient physicians were accepted as fact – Vesalius was one of the first to seek to prove or disprove their findings by his own work. In what seemed like blasphemy at the time, he was to prove Galen wrong on a number of counts. For example, he demonstrated that the mandible was made of only one bone and not two as Galen had thought.

Remarkably some surgeons continued to believe in Galen's writings – in spite of overwhelming evidence to the contrary.

Vesalius emphasised the active role of the learner in medical education: 'I strive that in public dissection the students do as much as possible so that if even the least trained of them must dissect a cadaver before a group of spectators, he will be able to perform it accurately with his own hands; and by comparing their studies one with another they will properly understand this part of medicine' (2).

Notes

1. Copyrighted work available under Creative Commons Attribution only licence CC BY 2.0, see http://creativecommons.org/licenses/by/2.0/.

2. *De Humani Corporis Fabrica Libri Septem*. 1543.

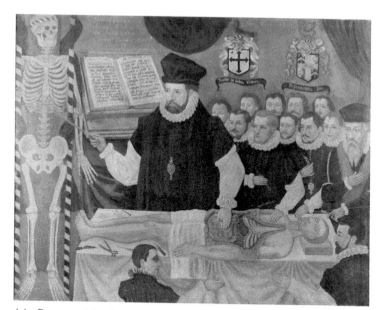

John Banester giving the visceral lecture at Barber-Surgeons' Hall, London, in 1581. Oil By: Anonymous, after Orr, Jack. (Credit: Wellcome Library [1].)

26 JOHN BANESTER GIVING THE VISCERAL LECTURE AT BARBER-SURGEONS' HALL

John Banester (1533–1610) was an English anatomist, teacher and surgeon. Perhaps following Hippocrates' dictum – 'he who desires to practice surgery must go to war' – he travelled on a military expedition to the continent (2). On his return, he gained a licence to practice medicine – albeit with the caveat that he should contact a colleague in cases of uncertainty. He passed on much that he had learned in Europe to his contemporaries, and was to show kindness to old soldiers for the rest of his career.

In this picture, Banester is adopting a multimedia approach to his presentation. He is palpating the viscera and pointing at a skeleton; behind him a textbook lays open. The learners in turn listen and watch intently; one places a hand on the body and another raises his hand as if to ask a question. In modern parlance, educational media should be 'discursive, adaptive, interactive and reflective' (3). Banester is certainly following this advice here.

Notes

1. Copyrighted work available under Creative Commons Attribution only licence CC BY 4.0, http://creativecommons.org/licenses/by/4.0/.

2. Corpus Hippocraticum, see https://archive.org/stream/hippocrates01hippuoft/ hippocrates01hippuoft_djvu.txt (accessed 9 March 2016).

3. Jamieson A. Future trends in e-learning. In Sandars J (Ed.), *E-Learning for GP Educators*. Oxon, UK: Radcliffe Publishing; 2006, pp. 137–144.

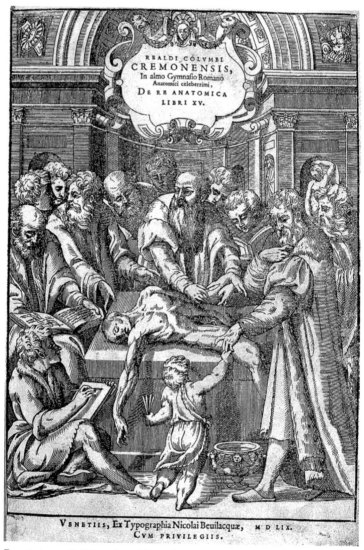

Frontispiece with illustration of dissection scene with anatomist demonstrating to an audience Woodcut 1559. From: De re anatomica libri XV/. By: Realdo Colombo. Published: N. Beuilacquæ, Venetiis: 1559. Title Page Size: (fol.). (Credit: Wellcome Library [1].)

27 DE RE ANATOMICA LIBRI XV, REALDO COLOMBO

Realdo Colombo (1516–1559) was an Italian anatomist and surgeon. He initially read philosophy in Milan, then studied to become an apothecary and finally took up anatomy and surgery at the University of Padua. His most important contribution to anatomy was the discovery of the pulmonary circulation. Before Colombo, it was thought that air was supplied to the heart by means of the pulmonary vein. However, Colombo correctly discovered that venous blood travelled from the heart to the lungs by the pulmonary artery and then returned as arterial blood by the pulmonary vein. These discoveries laid the foundations for William Harvey to build upon.

Colombo had a public feud with Vesalius. He drew attention to several mistakes in the latter's work, and in turn Vesalius personally criticised Colombo for his lack of knowledge. Feuds in medicine and medical education were to follow a similar pattern for centuries to come – with both sides having an unfortunate tendency to mix personalities, egos and science.

Colombo was a great believer in learning and teaching from practical experience (rather than simply learning from the ancients). 'A man learns more in a day by the dissection of a dog than by continually feeling the pulse and studying Galen's writing for many months together' (2).

Once again in this image there is no question but that the learners are part of the scene. They lean forward, read books, discuss among themselves and take notes.

Notes

1. Copyrighted work available under Creative Commons Attribution only licence CC BY 4.0, http://creativecommons.org/licenses/by/4.0.
2. Realdo Colombo. *De re anatomica libri*. Venet 1559. Lib XIV; 258.

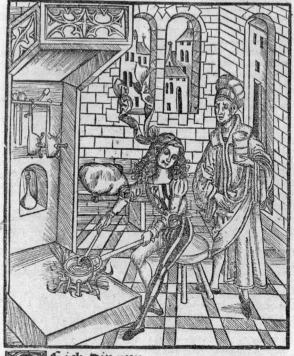

A physician in traditional costume holding an ointment jar is supervising an apprentice who is mixing a concoction in a pot over a fire. Woodcut Early Sixteenth Century. From: Spiegl der Artzny des gleichen vormals nie von keinem doctor in tütsch uszgangen ist nützlich und gutt allen denen so d'artzt radt begerent, auch den gestreiffelten leyen, welche sich und erwinden mit artznei umb zegon. In welchem du findst bericht aller hendel der artznei gezogen usz de fürnemsten büchern d'alten, mit schönen bewerten stucken und kurtz wyligen reden gemacht. By: Friesz, Laurent. Published: J. GrieningerStrassburg 1519. (Credit: Wellcome Library [1].)

28 A PHYSICIAN SUPERVISING AN APPRENTICE

Supervision has always been an important component of medical education. Beginners need close supervision and experts can practice unsupervised. The question has always been when and how to move from the first state to the second. What would patients think or want? Even that is not completely clear: Kenneth Wong asks, 'What does the patient think about a surgical trainee performing his first unsupervised appendectomy or his first unsupervised bowel resection? Yet, conversely does the patient want a fully qualified surgeon who has never operated unsupervised whilst training?' (2). What we can say for certain is that in the past trainee doctors practiced with too little supervision and the outcomes were harmful for both doctors and patients.

An important advance in medical education is improved educational and clinical supervision. Currently there is much interest in the transition of learners from the supervised to the unsupervised state. This transition is more complex than was once thought – it takes time and it depends on what exactly is the task at hand. For example, a trainee might be able to carry out an appendicectomy unsupervised but may not be able to carry out a cholecystectomy unsupervised.

This image shows an insightful take on supervision: the apprentice stirs the pot serenely while the supervisor peers anxiously over his shoulder. Is the apprentice reassured by the proximity of the supervisor? Is the supervisor about to intervene?

Notes

1. Copyrighted work available under Creative Commons Attribution only licence CC BY 4.0, http://creativecommons.org/licenses/by/4.0/.
2. Wong K. The ethics of medical training. *BMJ* (Published 9 August 2003).

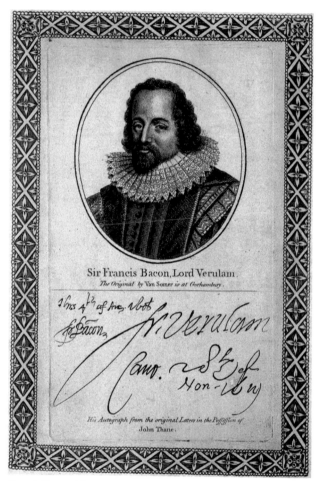

Francis Bacon, Viscount St Albans. Line engraving after van Somer. (Credit: Wellcome Library [1].)

29 FRANCIS BACON

Francis Bacon (1561–1626) was an English philosopher, scientist and writer. He was a champion of using the scientific method to advance knowledge and learning. His great work *Novum Organum* opens as follows: 'they who have presumed to dogmatize on nature, as on some well investigated subject, either from self-conceit or arrogance, and in the professorial style, have inflicted the greatest injury on philosophy and learning' (2). Bacon wanted to end dogma and build on science. However, he was critical of the methods of universities: 'again in the habits and regulations of schools, universities and the like assemblies, destined for the abode of learned men and the improvement of learning, everything is opposed to the progress of the sciences; for the lectures and exercises are so ordered, that anything out of the common track can scarcely enter the thoughts and contemplations of the mind' (2).

Bacon was apparently to die as he had lived: he apparently caught pneumonia while studying the effect of snow on the preservation of food. This at least is the account given by the author John Aubrey. This account is certainly compelling – the pre-enlightenment scholar travelling through London is suddenly inspired by the cold weather to conduct an experiment on the preservation of meat. However other accounts make no mention of the experiment. Who should we believe? Medical education needs narratives and stories and occasionally even legends. Sometimes 'when the legend becomes fact', it is best to 'print the legend'.

Notes

1. Copyrighted work available under Creative Commons Attribution only licence CC BY 2.0, see http://creativecommons.org/licenses/by/2.0.
2. Bacon F. *Organum Novum*. First book.

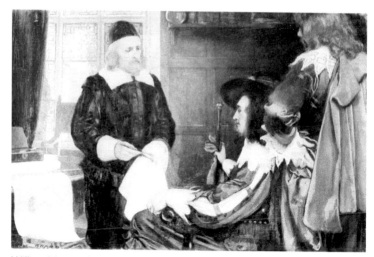

William Harvey demonstrating his theory of circulation of the blood before
Charles I. Oil painting by Ernest Board. (Credit: Wellcome Library [1].)

30 WILLIAM HARVEY DEMONSTRATING HIS THEORY OF CIRCULATION OF THE BLOOD

William Harvey (1578–1657) was an English physician who was among the first to describe the circulation of the blood. He conducted numerous experiments on animals to prove his theories and eventually published his findings in his treatise *On the Motion of the Heart and Blood*. Before Harvey, it was thought that the arterial and venous systems were largely separate and only came in contact through pores in the ventricles – these pores were invisible. However, Harvey correctly showed that the heart pumped blood into the arteries and that blood returned to the heart by means of veins. He was never able to show how blood passed from arteries to veins but suspected that small blood vessels must be enabling this passage.

Harvey lectured extensively on anatomy and also laid out tenets for what he saw as good practice in medical education. These included only going into as much detail as is necessary and making the best use of dissection and pathological demonstration in education: 'I profess both to learn and to teach anatomy, not from books but from dissections; not from positions of philosophers but from the fabric of nature' (2).

In this image, Harvey is standing and the learner is relaxing in his chair – this role-reversal seems surprising until you discover that the learner is King Charles I. Harvey was physician to Charles and to his father King James – indeed he dedicated his acclaimed treatise to Charles.

Notes

1. Copyrighted work available under Creative Commons Attribution only licence CC BY 2.0, see http://creativecommons.org/licenses/by/2.0/.
2. Dedication to Dr. Argent and Other Learned Physicians, see https://en.wikiquote.org/wiki/William_Harvey (accessed 9 March 2016).

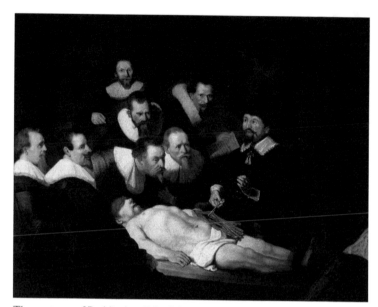

The anatomy of Dr. Nicolaes Tulp. Oil painting after Rembrandt van Rijn. By: Rembrandt Harmenszoon van Rijn. (Credit: Wellcome Library [1].)

31 THE ANATOMY LESSON OF DR. NICOLAES TULP

Nicolaes Tulp (1593–1674) was a Dutch surgeon. He was also a college tutor and performed anatomy demonstrations on criminals who had been executed. He was educated at the University of Leiden and on graduation rapidly grew a large practice in Amsterdam. He was also responsible for inspection of apothecaries in the city and drove up standards by publishing a pharmacopoeia.

Tulp was to be immortalised by Rembrandt in *The Anatomy Lesson of Dr. Nicolaes Tulp*. The picture is a masterpiece. It captures the excitement of discovery and brings to mind Bagehot's comment on history: 'The best history is but like the art of Rembrandt; it casts a vivid light on certain selected causes, on those which were best and greatest; it leaves all the rest in shadow and unseen' (2). The body is that of a robber – Aris Kindt (dissections were only legal if carried out on male criminals). The dissection has just begun on the cadaver's forearm, even though it is not clear why Tulp would have started there. It is no coincidence that the cadaver's face is partly in shadow – this was known as the shadow of death and was a signature technique of Rembrandt.

Notes

1. Copyrighted work available under Creative Commons Attribution only licence CC BY 2.0, see http://creativecommons.org/licenses/by/2.0/.
2. *Physics and Politics* (1872), Ch. 2, Sect. 2.

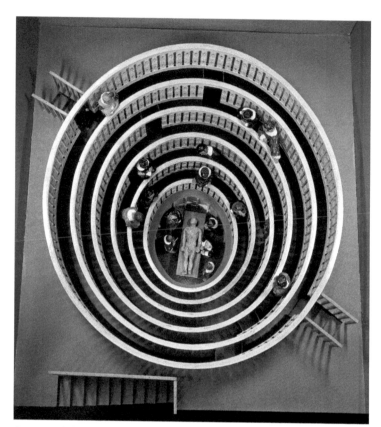

Anatomical theatre at Padua, Diorama. (Credit: Wellcome Library [1].)

32 ANATOMICAL THEATRE AT PADUA, DIORAMA

The anatomical theatre at Padua was built in 1594. Theatres were used to teach anatomy in early medical schools. Anatomical dissections took place in the centre, and the surrounding tiers enabled students to get a good view. The anatomical theatre at Padua was the first of its kind.

The University of Padua was founded in 1222 when a group of free-thinking academics and their students splintered from the University of Bologna. This spirit of scientific freedom was encapsulated in the university motto: *Universa Universis Patavina Libertas* (Paduan freedom is universal for everyone). This freedom attracted scholars from around the world – alumni of the medical school were to include Andreas Vesalius, Realdo Colombo and William Harvey (Images 25, 27 and 30 in this book). Others included Giovanni Battista Morgagni and Bernardino Ramazzini (1682–1771). Morgagni was professor of anatomy at the school and is credited with developing the concept that diseases in body organs result in clinical manifestations. Ramazzini (1633–1714) was professor of theoretical medicine and was the first to describe occupational diseases in various workers.

The anatomical theatre was the centre of the medical school, and anatomy was to be the foundation of medical education for the next several hundred years. As Henry Morris claimed in 1876, 'if the physician be ignorant of anatomy, how is he to diagnose disease?' (2).

Notes

1. Copyrighted work available under Creative Commons Attribution only licence CC BY 2.0, see http://creativecommons.org/licenses/by/2.0/.
2. Morris H. A lecture introductory to the course on anatomy. *BMJ* 1876;2:515.

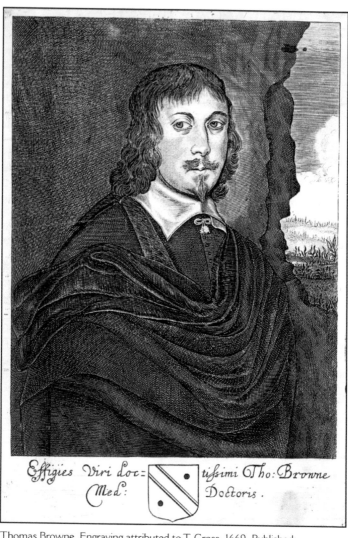

Thomas Browne. Engraving attributed to T. Cross, 1669. Published: London, 1669. (Credit: Wellcome Library [1].)

33 THOMAS BROWNE

Thomas Browne (1605–1682) was an English writer, physician and scientist. In his books, he commonly debunked received wisdom in medicine – but always in a light and engaging style. He was also a voracious reader and an early champion of lifelong learning: 'I keepe the sheets of the transactions [of the Royal Society] as they come out monethly' (2). Browne started his medical studies at Oxford and then travelled to Padua and Montpellier before attaining his degree in Leiden. Two of Browne's most noted publications include *Religio Medici* (The Religion of a Physician) and *Pseudodoxia Epidemica* (Enquiries into Very Many Received Tenets and Commonly Presumed Truths).

Pseudodoxia Epidemica offers much insight into Browne's thoughts on education. According to Browne, 'this is one reason why, though Universities be full of men, they are oftentimes empty of learning: Why, as there are some men do much without learning, so others but little with it, and few that attain to any measure of it. For many heads that undertake it, were never squared, nor timber'd for it' (3). Browne was also forthright about the need to continually question received wisdom and remain flexible in our thinking and beliefs, and to be always ready to review our thoughts in light of new knowledge or reasoning (3).

Notes

1. Copyrighted work available under Creative Commons Attribution only licence CC BY 2.0, see http://creativecommons.org/licenses/by/2.0/.

2. Shaw AB. Sir Thomas Browne: The man and the physician. *BMJ* 1982;285:40.

3. http://www.gutenberg.org/files/39960/39960-h/39960-h.htm#PSEUDODOXIA_EPIDEMICA (accessed 20 April 2015).

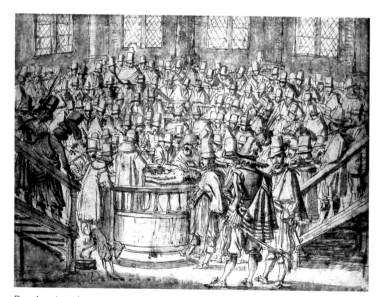

Pen drawing: the anatomy theatre at Leiden during a dissection. Seventeenth century. By: Willem Buytenwegh. (Credit: Wellcome Library [I].)

34 DISSECTION AT THE ANATOMY THEATRE AT LEIDEN

The University of Leiden was founded in 1575 by William, Prince of Orange, and the medical school at the university became a powerhouse of medical education during the eighteenth century. Boerhaave was one of the main driving forces behind the university. Boerhaave was first and foremost a teacher, and the culture of learning attracted students from around the world.

According to Olle ten Cate, this culture remains in Dutch medical education to this day. 'The open and relatively tolerant Dutch culture, slightly scared from traditions and regulations, makes a fertile soil for investigation, experimentation and improvement of medical education, in a way that might have surprised Boerhaave – but he would have liked it, had he lived now instead of in the Golden Age?' (2) The Dutch Golden Age was an era of Dutch supremacy in military, economic and financial affairs, and also in philosophic and scientific matters. According to Bertrand Russell, 'it is impossible to exaggerate the importance of Holland in the seventeenth century, as the one country where there was freedom of speculation' (3).

This drawing shows much theatre but maybe not as much learning as it could. Some learners are far too back to see and some are looking at the artist. An emaciated dog wanders around the foreground.

Notes

1. Copyrighted work available under Creative Commons Attribution only licence CC BY 2.0, see http://creativecommons.org/licenses/by/2.0.

2. ten Cate O. Medical education in the Netherlands. *Med Teach* 2007;29(8):752–757.

3. Russell B. *A History of Western Philosophy*, George Allen & Unwin Ltd, London, 1945.

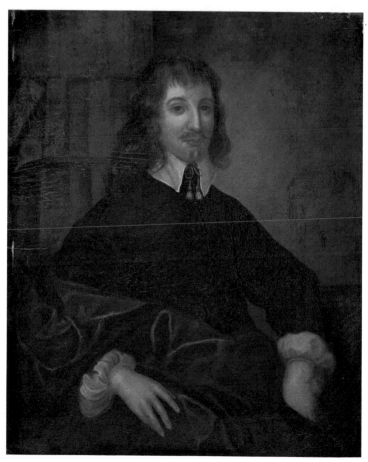

Nicolas Culpeper. Oil painting. (Credit: Wellcome Library [1].)

35 NICOLAS CULPEPER

Nicholas Culpeper (1616–1654) was an English physician, herbalist and astrologer. He wrote three books including *The English Physician, Complete Herbal* and *Astrological Judgement of Diseases from the Decumbiture of the Sick*. He believed in natural medicine and was critical of the artificial and expensive treatments prescribed by contemporary physicians. He believed that his colleagues were too ready to follow tradition and too often unwilling to reason or experiment. He married into a wealthy family and simply collected his herbal remedies from the fields around Spitalfields in east London – this enabled him to provide services to patients for free. He felt that many of his fellow physicians were motivated by greed and he was forthright in saying so. His opinions made him unpopular amongst the medical hierarchy but he remained outspoken until his early death from tuberculosis: 'For God's sake build not your faith upon Tradition, 'tis as rotten as a rotten Post' (2). Culpeper was equally critical of lawyers and priests.

This portrait shows a young, fresh-faced, idealistic Culpeper – well before tuberculosis would have taken hold.

Notes

1. Copyrighted work available under Creative Commons Attribution only licence CC BY 2.0, see http://creativecommons.org/licenses/by/2.0/.

2. http://www.brainyquote.com/quotes/authors/n/nicholas_culpeper.html (accessed 10 March 2014).

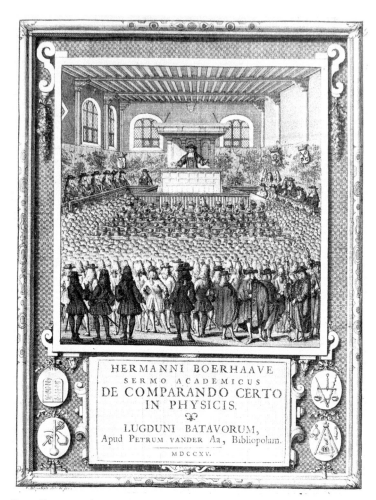

From: Sermo academicus de comparando certo in physicis. Published: P. van der AaLeiden, 1715. (Credit: Wellcome Library [1].)

36 BOERHAAVE GIVING A LECTURE

Herman Boerhaave (1668–1738) was a Dutch physician and medical educator. He was professor of botany and medicine at the university of Leiden and reformed medical instruction there. He described Boerhaave syndrome – tearing of the oesophagus caused by vomiting.

According to Andrew MacPhail, 'Boerhaave lectured five hours a day; his hospital contained only twelve beds, but by Sydenham's method he made of it the medical centre of Europe' (2). Boerhaave was most famous as a teacher and he clearly had high standards. Here is Boerhaave on his contemporary physicians: 'If we compare the good which a half dozen true sons of Aesculapius have accomplished since the origin of medical art upon the earth, with the evil which the immense mass of doctors of this profession among the human race have done, there can be no doubt that it would have been far better if there had never been any physicians in the world' (3).

This image shows Boerhaave in his prime delivering a lecture at Leiden. The image comes from the title page of one of his books. Boerhaave's lectures became famous and attracted learners from around Europe. This image is clearly intended to show the greatness of Boerhaave. He is not only elevated above his learners, he also appears physically larger than them. His dress and body habitus all suggest the power of a man who was a physical and intellectual colossus.

Notes

1. Copyrighted work available under Creative Commons Attribution only licence CC BY 2.0, see http://creativecommons.org/licenses/by/2.0/.

2. MacPhail A. An address on the source of modern medicine. *BMJ* 1933;1(3767): 443–447.

3. Tan SY, Hu M. Hermann Boerhaave (1668–1738): 18th century teacher extraordinaire. *Singapore Med J* 2004;45(1):3–5.

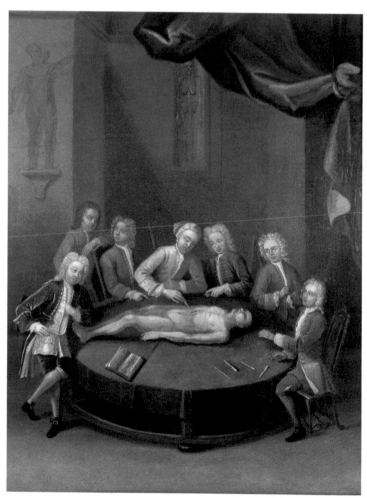

William Cheselden giving an anatomical demonstration to six spectators in the anatomy theatre of the Barber-Surgeons' Company, London. Oil painting, ca. 1730/1740. (Credit: Wellcome Library [1].)

37 WILLIAM CHESELDEN GIVING AN ANATOMICAL DEMONSTRATION

William Cheselden (1688–1752) was an English anatomist and surgeon. He published two books – *Anatomy of the Human Body* and *The Anatomy of Bones*. Both were to become seminal texts in medical education. He championed practical anatomy and was critical of those who by 'dividing and describing the parts, more than the knowledge of their uses requires, perplexes the learner, and makes the science dry, and difficult' (2). Both books were published in the English language – which was revolutionary at the time; before them most medical books were published only in Latin. Their accessibility to English readers undoubtedly contributed to their popularity. The elegance of the images in both books also attracted a wide readership. Cheselden realised the utility of the image and its advantages over text. In the preface to *The Anatomy of Bones*, he writes: 'I thought it useless to make long descriptions, one view of such prints shewing more than the fullest and best description can possibly do'.

Cheselden encouraged the break between the barbers and surgeons – he felt that surgical science was being held back by this relationship. He helped found the Company of Surgeons in 1745 – this would eventually become the Royal College of Surgeons.

This picture must have predated the break with the barbers – the location is the anatomy theatre of the Barber-Surgeons' Company. Most striking about the picture is the learners and the various activities they are undertaking – observing, listening and discussing.

Notes

1. Copyrighted work available under Creative Commons Attribution only licence CC BY 2.0, see http://creativecommons.org/licenses/by/2.0/.
2. https://archive.org/stream/anatomyofhumanbo1750ches#page/n9/mode/2up (accessed 9 March 2016).

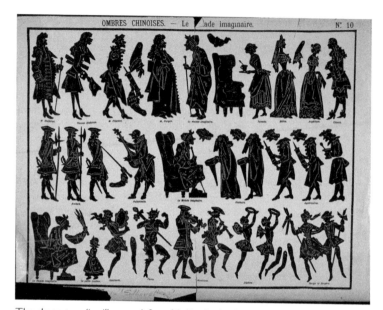

The characters (in silhouette) from Molière's play *La malade imaginaire*. Process print. After: Jean-Baptiste Poquelin de Molière. (Credit: Wellcome Library [I].)

38 THE CHARACTERS (IN SILHOUETTE) FROM MOLIÈRE'S PLAY *LA MALADE IMAGINAIRE*

Le Malade imaginaire is a three-act comedy by Molière. It was first performed in 1673 in Paris. It is a satire on society, medicine and medical education. In this quote, the character Mr Diafoirus, a physician, talks about his son Thomas, a medical student: 'he never showed signs of a lively imagination, nor of a quick intelligence you find in some; but these were qualities which led me to forsee that his judgement would be strong, a quality essential to the exercise of our art…Eventually after much hard slog, he succeeded in graduating with glory; and I can say without vanity that in his two years on the benches, no candidate has made more noise than he in the disputes of our school. He has made himself formidable, and no thesis can be advanced without his arguing the opposite case to its ultimate extreme' (2).

The play satirises physicians' greed, vanity, ignorance and lack of caring. This print portrays the grotesque energy of the characters – an achievement considering they are in silhouette. Ironically Molière collapsed on stage while playing the hypochondriac in *Le malade imaginaire*. He had a pulmonary haemorrhage caused by tuberculosis and died within hours.

Notes

1. Copyrighted work available under Creative Commons Attribution only licence CC BY 2.0, 1673, see http://creativecommons.org/licenses.
2. Moliere JP. *Le Malade Imaginaire*, see http://www.gutenberg.org/files/9070/9070-h/9070-h.htm (accessed 9 March 2016).

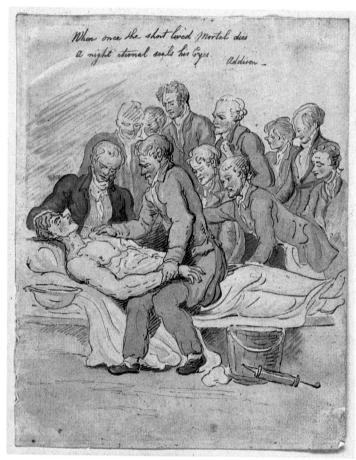

A group of doctors and medical students surround a dying patient. Watercolour painting. (Credit: Wellcome Library [1].)

39 A GROUP OF DOCTORS AND MEDICAL STUDENTS SURROUND A DYING PATIENT

According to Denis Hill, 'Medical education is not without its pains and its anxieties. The realities of disease and death are themselves painful and often shocking' (2).

Medical educators have always struggled to introduce the tangible realities of death and dying to medical students and junior doctors. Most doctors can remember the first person who died while under their care – so their experiences in this regard are likely to be vivid learning experiences. However, the dilemma lies in whether and how to teach palliative care at the bedside. How do you balance the need for privacy and dignity of the patient and family with the practical learning needs of the students?

This picture shows a dying patient surrounded by a group of doctors and medical students. However, the picture is as notable as much for what is missing as for what is present. Where is the patient's family? Where are the nurses? On the other hand, perhaps a welcome absence is the lack of intravenous lines, intubation equipment, cardiorespiratory monitors and other modern sacramental instruments of death and dying. The inscription at the top of the image reads

When once the short lived mortal dies
A night eternal seals his eyes.

Notes

1. Copyrighted work available under Creative Commons Attribution only licence CC BY 2.0, see http://creativecommons.org/licenses/by/2.0/.
2. Hill D. Acceptance of psychiatry by the medical student. *BMJ* 1960;1:917.

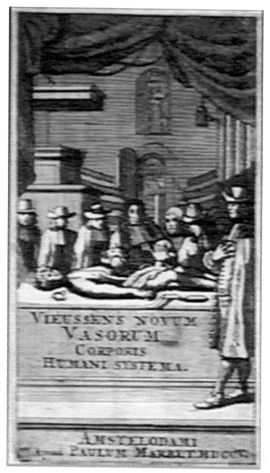

An anatomical dissection with six onlookers and the dissector who is retracting the skin to reveal the intestines. Engraving, 1705. After: Raymond de Vieussens. Published: Apud Paulum Marret, Amstelodami [Amsterdam]. (Credit: Wellcome Library [1].)

40 AN ANATOMICAL DISSECTION WITH SIX ONLOOKERS AND THE DISSECTOR WHO IS RETRACTING THE SKIN TO REVEAL THE INTESTINES

'I strive that in public dissection the students do as much as possible so that if even the least trained of them must dissect a cadaver before a group of spectators, he will be able to perform it accurately with his own hands; and by comparing their studies one with another they will properly understand this part of medicine'.

Andreas Vesalius (2)

Learning by dissection was a core component of medical education for centuries. Today there is ongoing debate about the role of cadaveric dissection in education. Certainly it encourages observational and self-directed learning skills. It also enables the development of dissection skills themselves, although the effectiveness of its role in this regard has been questioned. According to Collins, 'dissection of cadavers is expensive, time consuming, and emotionally disturbing for some students', and 'the preserved tissues don't always provide an accurate impression of the living body' (3). As with most methods of medical education, its effectiveness depends on the context of use. It is likely to be helpful for those in postgraduate training in surgery but less helpful for medical students.

In this image, the learners are involved and close to the action – but it is not clear who the figure at the front is. Is he a guard keeping an eye out for intruders? Or is he the teacher – instructing both the dissector and the students?

Notes

1. Copyrighted work available under Creative Commons Attribution only licence CC BY 2.0, see http://creativecommons.org/licenses/by/2.0.

2. *De Humani Corporis Fabrica Libri Septem*, 1543, see http://www.e-rara.ch/bau_1/content/titleinfo/6299027 (accessed 9 March 2016).

3. Collins J. Modern approaches to teaching and learning anatomy. *BMJ* 2008;337:a1310.

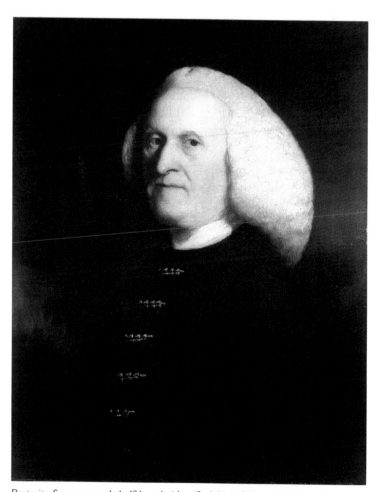

Portrait of a man, nearly half-length, identified doubtfully with William Hunter; attributed to Joshua Reynolds, dated on reverse '1782'. (Credit: Wellcome Library [1].)

41 WILLIAM HUNTER

William Hunter (1718–1783) was a Scottish physician, obstetrician and medical teacher. His passion was communicating his knowledge to others and he was keen to introduce European ideas to British medicine. He did his initial training in anatomy at St George's Hospital and subsequently went on to become one of the most acclaimed obstetricians in London.

His thoughts on how best to educate a physician – 'Were I to place a man of proper talents, in the most direct road for becoming truly great in his profession, I would chuse a good practical anatomist, and put him into a large hospital to attend the sick, and dissect the dead' (2). Certainly there is no questioning his commitment to medicine and to medical education. It is said of him that 'he worked till he dropped and he lectured when he was dying' (3). Hunter left his collections to the University of Glasgow where they are now housed in the Hunterian Museum. The purpose of his bequest was to assist the students of the university in their learning. This painting is by Joshua Reynolds, an eighteenth-century portrait painter and the first president of the Royal Academy.

Notes

1. Copyrighted work available under Creative Commons Attribution only licence CC BY 2.0, see http://creativecommons.org/licenses/by/2.0/.
2. *Last Course of Anatomical Lectures*, Lecture 2, see https://archive.org/details/b21441145 (accessed 9 March 2016).
3. Garrison FH. *An Introduction to the History of Medicine*. Saunders: Philadelphia, PA; 1914.

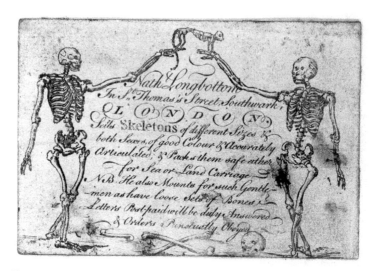

Trade-card of Nathaniel Longbottom, supplier of skeletons, St Thomas's Street, Southwark. (Credit: Wellcome Library [1].)

42 TRADE-CARD OF NATHANIEL LONGBOTTOM, SUPPLIER OF SKELETONS

This image is the trade-card of Nathaniel Longbottom, a supplier of skeletons, in St Thomas's Street, Southwark. The trade-card was likely to have been printed in the mid-eighteenth century – although the exact date is not known. The card claims that Longbottom will supply skeletons of different sizes and both sexes and that they are of good colour and accurately articulated. It is likely that he was supplying them to medical students and local medical schools; however, the card also promises that they can be packed safe either for sea or land carriage.

Longbottom appears a man of entrepreneurial spirit and meticulous efficiency; he will mount for gentlemen who have loose sets of bones and will punctually obey orders. Much of his custom likely came from the nearby St Thomas' Hospital. This was probably the destination of most of the skeletons, but how Longbottom came to acquire them is unknown.

The design of the card is imaginative – skeletons with arms raised above a section of text and supporting the skeleton of a monkey. However the tone of the text is deferential, almost servile. Longbottom is clearly a man of trade and must show humility when dealing with gentleman physicians or would-be physicians. It would be interesting to see the prices, but mentioning money was perhaps considered too crude.

Note

1. Copyrighted work available under Creative Commons Attribution only licence CC BY 4.0, http://creativecommons.org/licenses/by/4.0/.

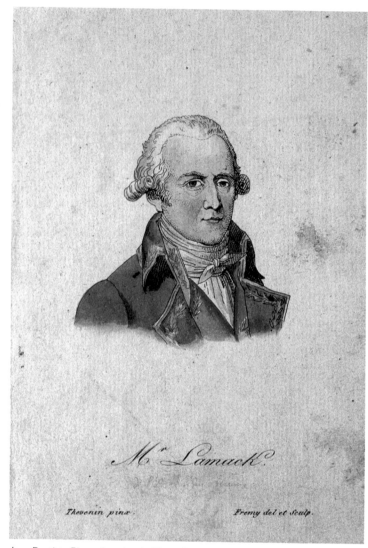

Jean Baptiste Pierre Antoine de Monet Lamarck. Coloured etching by J. M. Frémy after C. Thévenin, 180. (Credit: Wellcome Library [1].)

43 LAMARCK

Jean Baptiste Pierre Antoine de Monet Lamarck (1744–1829) was a French academic, scholar and biologist. Lamarck started life as a soldier in the French army and impressed his seniors with his physical and moral courage. However, an illness forced an early retirement from the army, so he decided to study medicine and then botany and biology. Lamarck carefully navigated the politics of the French revolution and was appointed professor of invertebrate zoology at the National Museum of Natural History in Paris.

His work was to leave a lasting legacy on both biology and medicine. He published extensively on the classification of invertebrates and on the inheritance of acquired characteristics. He was always keen not only to discover but to pass on his learning and discoveries to others: 'It is not enough to discover and prove a useful truth previously unknown, but that it is necessary also to be able to propagate it and get it recognized' (2).

Today Lamarck remains a figure of some controversy among students of biology, evolution and indeed of medical history. Some historians feel that a myth about Lamarck has been built up, and that 'misrepresentations of Lamarck form part of a bigger folly: Textbooks pit Lamarck against Darwin in a mythical contest from which Darwin emerges victorious' (3). The simple truth may be that medicine and medical education need stories and some stories are elaborated in order to convey a message.

Notes

1. Copyrighted work available under Creative Commons Attribution only licence CC BY 2.0, see http://creativecommons.org/licenses/by/2.0/.
2. *Philosophie Zoologique*, 1809, see http://www.goodreads.com/quotes/979655-it-is-not-enough-to-discover-and-prove-a-useful (accessed 9 March 2016).
3. http://www.textbookleague.org/54marck.htm (accessed 6 April 2015).

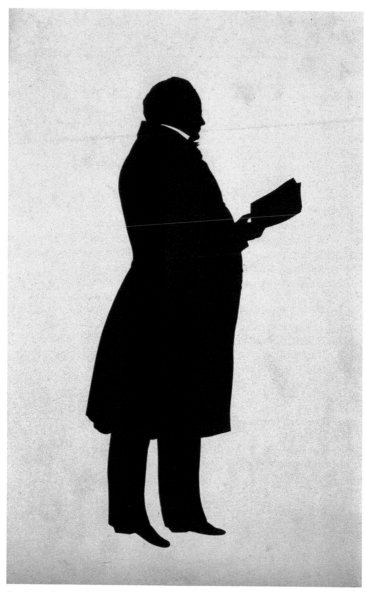

Sir Astley Paston Cooper. Silhouette. (Credit: Wellcome Library [1].)

44 ASTLEY PASTON COOPER

Astley Paston Cooper (1768–1841) was an English surgeon and anatomist. He lectured at the Royal College of Surgeons and was surgeon to three consecutive monarchs. He discovered a range of diseases and anatomical structures – from Cooper's disease (breast cysts) to Cooper's ligaments (the ligaments of the breast). A dedicated teacher and learner, he claimed that there was 'no short road to knowledge' and was willing to admit his mistakes: 'I have made many mistakes myself; in learning the anatomy of the eye I dare say, I have spoiled a hatfull; the best surgeon, like the best general, is he who makes the fewest mistakes' (2).

This willingness to admit and learn from mistakes was unusual at the time and was to remain so for another 150 years. However the modern quality improvement movement in healthcare has helped transform the culture of medicine. The first step in quality improvement is recognising that there is a problem with quality and auditing the problems (3). Following this, efforts to improve quality can begin. Cooper also guided his colleagues to always put themselves in the place of the patient when making decisions: 'in the performance of our duty one feeling should direct us; the case we should consider as our own, and we should ask ourselves, whether, placed under similar circumstances, we should choose to submit to the pain and danger we are about to inflict' (4).

Notes

1. Copyrighted work available under Creative Commons Attribution only licence CC BY 2.0, see http://creativecommons.org/licenses/by/2.0.

2. *Fraser's Magazine* (Nov. 1862), 66, 574.

3. Walsh K, Gompertz PH, Rudd AG. Stroke care: How do we measure quality? *Postgrad Med J* 2002;78(920):322–326.

4. Cooper BB. *The Life of Sir Astley Cooper*, Vol. 2. 1843, p. 207.

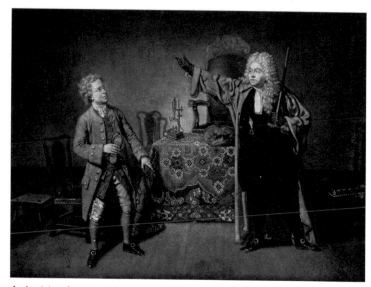

A physician shouting at his assistant. Mezzotint. (Credit: Wellcome Library [1].)

45 A PHYSICIAN SHOUTING AT HIS ASSISTANT

Here is a scene that we might hope to have consigned to history – a physician shouting at his assistant. If not, then these two quotes might help convince the unconvinced of the futility of bullying and the harm that it does. First, John Collier on why bullying doesn't help: 'bullying, intimidation, and humiliation are essential in maintaining all hierarchies, but I still can't find the evidence that they are any good for producing doctors' (2). Second, Diana Wood on harms: 'The negative impact that bullying and harassment have on the wellbeing of students and doctors, overall morale in the medical workforce, and recruitment and retention in the profession demand our continuing efforts to resolve these problems' (3).

Unfortunately bullying in medicine and medical education has not yet been consigned to the history books – it remains a significant problem to this day. Medical students and doctors in training are typically the victims of bullying. Hierarchical medical structures probably contribute to bullying – as does the bullying cycle where the bullied student eventually turns into the bullying senior.

In this print, the assistant is scared but also confused. He is unlikely to learn or to carry out the instructions asked of him.

Notes

1. Copyrighted work available under Creative Commons Attribution only licence CC BY 2.0, see http://creativecommons.org/licenses/by/2.0/.
2. Collier J. Personal view. Medical education as abuse. *BMJ* 1989;299:1408.
3. Wood DF. Bullying and harassment in medical schools. *BMJ* 2006;333:664.

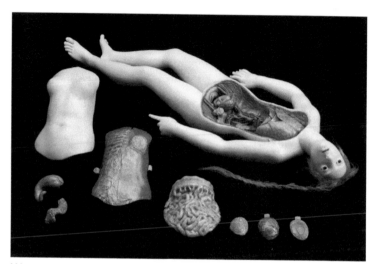

Wax anatomical figure of reclining woman, Florence, Italy. Maker: Susini, Clemente. Made: 1771–1800. (Credit: Science Museum, London, Wellcome Images [1].)

46 WAX ANATOMICAL FIGURE OF A RECLINING WOMAN

Wax anatomical figures were used in medical education in the seventeenth and eighteenth centuries. They were typically male, and female figures emphasised how the female body was different. Certainly the study of anatomy (by whatever means) was to dominate medical education for many centuries. By the twentieth century, some were beginning to question the clinical usefulness of this education: 'Many teachers of anatomy, physiology, and pathology (and perhaps this obtains more particularly at the universities devoid of clinical schools) instruct their students as though they, too, were destined to become anatomists, physiologists, and pathologists, whereas nine out of ten of them are destined to be doctors'. (2)

This anatomical model is fascinating. Its purpose was medical education but it prompts a number of questions: Why did it have hair? Why such piercing eyes? And why the pose? Models of this kind have intrigued and disturbed viewers for centuries. Their purpose was not only to educate but to cause wonder. The models are reclining, serene and, some think, alluring – or that they would be if their inner anatomy were not exposed. The models were created by Clemente Michelangelo Susini, an Italian sculptor. His models were based on partly dissected corpses.

Notes

1. Copyrighted work available under Creative Commons Attribution only licence CC BY 4.0, http://creativecommons.org/licenses/by/4.0/.
2. Ryle JA. The student in irons. *BMJ* 1932;1:587.

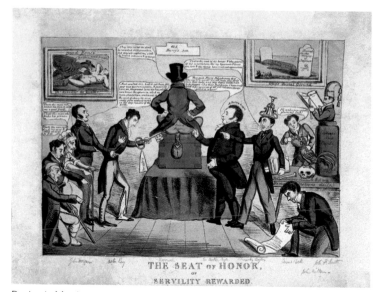

Benjamin Harrison, autocratic treasurer of Guy's Hospital, backing the gross nepotism of Sir Astley Cooper. Coloured lithograph by R. Cruikshank? 1830. (Credit: Wellcome Library [1].)

47 BENJAMIN HARRISON, AUTOCRATIC TREASURER OF GUY'S HOSPITAL

Benjamin Harrison (1771–1856) was treasurer of Guy's Hospital. He was 'viewed as an autocratic, even a despotic, administrator by contemporaries who referred to him as King Harrison' (2). However, he was a driving force behind the success of the medical school and oversaw a rapid expansion in its size and power. Was he one of the first people to realise the importance of funding streams for medical education? Certainly, Thomas Clifford Allbutt, writing nearly a century later, was keen to press the point home: 'but let it be clearly understood that all these betterments of medical education will cost money, and let us not hesitate to say so' (3).

In modern times, the growing cost of medical education has led to a renewed interest in ensuring that students, institutions and funders glean maximum return from their investments (4). The first step in this regard is ensuring that all the costs related to medical education are accounted for and that educational institutions are transparent about where the funds are spent. Then appropriate cost analyses must be applied to the educational endeavour – these might be cost effectiveness analyses, cost benefit analyses, cost utility analyses or cost feasibility analyses.

This lithograph shows the treasurer in his pomp: sitting on his chest and studiously ignoring the supplicants that surround him.

Notes

1. Copyrighted work available under Creative Commons Attribution only licence CC BY 2.0, see http://creativecommons.org/licenses/by/2.0.
2. http://www.oxforddnb.com/templates/article.jsp?articleid=12431&back=,12432 (accessed 10 March 2014).
3. Allbutt TC. Medical Education in England: A Note on Sir George Newman's Memorandum to the President of the Board of Education. *BMJ* 1918;2:113.
4. Walsh K, Rutherford A, Richardson J, Moore P. NICE medical education modules: An analysis of cost-effectiveness. *Educ Prim Care* 2010;21(6):396.

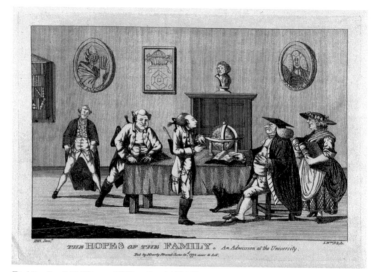

Etching by J. Williams, 1772, after H.W. Bunbury. Published: M Darly, [London] (Strand): accord to Act. 10 June 1772. (Credit: Wellcome Library [1].)

48 AN INCOMPETENT ENTRANT PRESENTED BY HIS FATHER TO A UNIVERSITY DIGNITARY

How best to select applicants for medical school is something that has puzzled the profession for many years. A variety of methods have been trialled – both singly and in combination. These have included structured interviews, tests of cognitive ability, personality tests, situational judgement tests, multiple mini-interviews, selection centres and the taking up of references. All have advantages and disadvantages in terms of the criteria of reliability, validity, feasibility or cost and acceptability to candidates.

And what have we learned? Certainly McKeown is correct in saying that 'it is easier to criticise the present selection procedure than to design a better one' (2). However, we have also come to realise the importance of selection. Henry Dicks has asked 'must it always be only in rueful valedictory repentance that the gatekeepers of medical education come to see what they have been doing' (3). Ultimately a programmatic approach to selection is likely to be the best practice. And long-term follow-up studies should enable us to find out more about the predictive capability of assessment methods.

The route of entry suggested in this image is unlikely to be predictive, programmatic or best practice. The etching is by Henry William Bunbury, an English caricaturist.

Notes

1. Copyrighted work available under Creative Commons Attribution only licence CC BY 4.0, http://creativecommons.org/licenses/by/4.0.
2. McKeown T. Personal view. *BMJ* 1986;293:200.
3. Dicks HV. Medical education and medical practice. *BMJ* 1965;2:818.

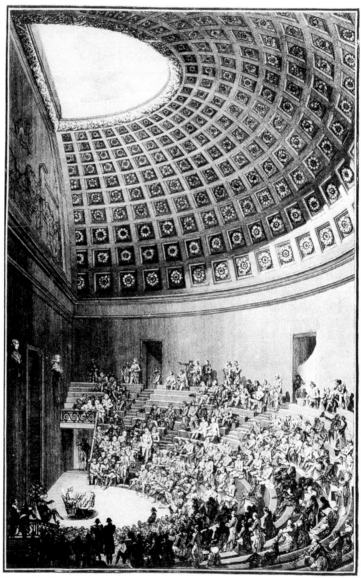

Ecole de chirurgie, Paris, scene in theatre showing anatomical demonstration. From: Description des ecoles de chirurgie. By: Jaques Gondoin. Published: P.D. Pierres Paris. 1780. Plate XXIX. (Credit: Wellcome Library [1].)

49 ECOLE DE CHIRURGIE, PARIS: ANATOMY THEATRE

The School of Surgery in Paris opened in 1774. It is most famous for its hemispherical amphitheatre, where anatomical dissections and lectures took place. This was designed by Jacques Gondouin, a French architect and designer. It could seat up to 1200 people and was open to members of the public as well as medical students. The school helped cement the reputation of Paris as a centre of excellence in medical education. The standard set was seen as a goal for other schools to aspire to: According to William Hunter, 'Gentlemen may have an opportunity of learning the art of dissecting during the whole winter season, in the same manner as at Paris' (2).

This image conveys the size and atmosphere of the amphitheatre – it feels like a cathedral of anatomy. According to Gondouin, the building is 'a monument of the beneficence of the King…which should have the character of magnificence relative to its function; a school whose fame attracts a great concourse of pupils from all nations should appear open and easy of access' (3).

Today the building is part of the headquarters of the Paris Descartes University.

Notes

1. Copyrighted work available under Creative Commons Attribution only licence CC BY 2.0, see http://creativecommons.org/licenses/by/2.0/.
2. Tweedy J. The Hunterian Oration: Delivered before the Royal College of Surgeons of England, February 14th, 1905. *BMJ* 1905;1:341.
3. Braham A. *The Architecture of the French Enlightenment*. Berkeley, CA: University of California Press; 1980.

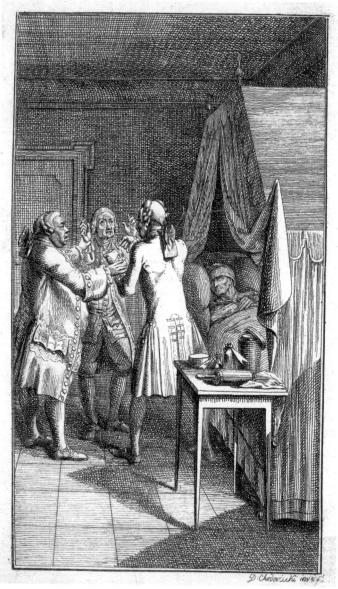

Doctors disputing, the patient is ignored. Etching by D.N. Chodowiecki, 1781. Published: s.n., Leipzig. 1781. (Credit: Wellcome Library [1].)

50 DOCTORS DISPUTING, THE PATIENT IS IGNORED

'Let the young know they will never find a more interesting, more instructive book than the patient himself'.

Giorgio Baglivi (2)

In modern medical education, patients can be instructors, facilitators, leaders, advisers, curriculum designers and much more. Medicine and medical education have everything to gain from their input. The question for medical educators is no longer whether patients should be involved, but how they should be involved and how barriers to close involvement can be overcome.

First of all patients must be recruited to the education team – ideally patients should be representative of the local population that doctors care for. Patients who have been recruited need preparation so that they are able to perform the tasks that have been asked of them. Many will need ongoing support after the initial period of preparation has been completed. Finally, many patients appreciate some form of recognition of their involvement in medical education. This might be in the form of payments but might equally be of a non-monetary kind – for example through special certificates.

Disputing doctors who ignore their patients should become museum pieces, and patients should become partners – both in medical education and in clinical care.

Notes

1. Copyrighted work available under Creative Commons Attribution only licence CC BY 2.0, see http://creativecommons.org/licenses/by/2.0.
2. http://medicalstate.tumblr.com/post/6597839959/let-the-young-know-they-will-never-find-a-more (accessed 9 March 2016).

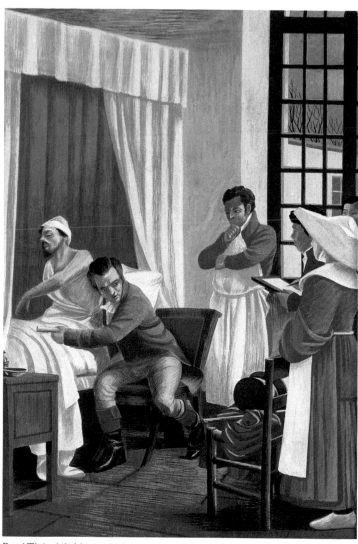

René Théophile Hyacinthe Laënnec auscultating a tuberculous patient at the Necker Hospital, Paris. Gouache after T. Chartran. (Credit: Wellcome Library [1].)

51 LAËNNEC

René Théophile Hyacinthe Laënnec (1781–1826) was a French physician and inventor of the stethoscope. Before Laënnec, physicians listened to the heart and lungs by pressing their ear directly against the chest wall. This was embarrassing when examining women and less than effective when examining overweight patients. Laënnec's stethoscope overcame both problems. His original apparatus was a cylinder – the physician held one end against the chest and the other against his ear. Laënnec was the first to use the terms 'rhonchi' and 'crepitance' when diagnosing respiratory conditions. He was professor of medicine at the Collège de France. Laënnec died of tuberculosis at the age of just 45 and left his personal stethoscope to a relative – describing it as 'the greatest legacy of my life' (2).

Here is Laënnec auscultating a patient with tuberculosis. The painting is by Theobold Chartran – a French propaganda painter. There is no question but that Chartran has conveyed a message in the painting: the patient is grey, thin, almost lifeless. By contrast, Laënnec is energetic and full of the enthusiasm of discovery. A small team stand close by – all eyes on the great man.

The enthusiasm of discovery can also be found in Laënnec's own description of the first time he used his apparatus when examining a young woman: 'Taking a sheet of paper I rolled it into a very tight roll, one end of which I placed on the precordial region, whilst I put my ear to the other. I was both surprised and gratified at being able to hear the beating of the heart with much greater clearness and distinctness than I had ever before by direct application of my ear' (3).

Notes

1. Copyrighted work available under Creative Commons Attribution only licence CC BY 2.0, see http://creativecommons.org/licenses/by/2.0/.
2. http://en.wikipedia.org/wiki/Ren%C3%A9_Laennec (accessed 9 March 2016).
3. Porter R. *The Cambridge Illustrated History of Medicine*. Cambridge University Press: Cambridge, UK; 2001, pp. 173–174.

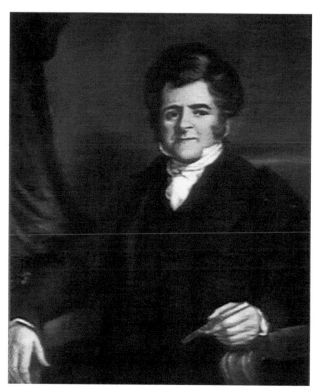

Richard Bright (1789–1858), physician. Oil painting after Frederick Richard Say. (Credit: Wellcome Library [1].)

52 RICHARD BRIGHT

Richard Bright (1789–1858) was an English physician, educator and researcher. He conducted research into kidney disease at Guy's Hospital and discovered nephritis – originally called Bright's disease. Contemporaries at Guy's included Thomas Addison and Thomas Hodgkin. Bright was a dedicated teacher and encouraged his students to always place their patients at the centre of their learning: 'Acute disease must be seen at least once a day by those who wish to learn; in many cases twice a day will not be too often' (2).

One criticism of modern medical education is that it no longer holds to Bright's recommendation. Both undergraduate students and postgraduate trainees (and their tutors) complain that they do not follow up sufficient numbers of patients and so cannot learn the natural history of the disease. Longitudinal integrated clerkships are a recent attempt to overcome this problem. Longitudinal integrated clerkships enable students to follow patients from the start to the end of their illness. The idea is to give a broader view of healthcare and to help students develop long-term relationships with patients and their families. Bright would likely have approved.

This rather formal and posed painting was by Frederick Richard Say. Say was primarily a portrait painter, but also drew images of pathological specimens for Bright.

Notes

1. Copyrighted work available under Creative Commons Attribution only licence CC BY 2.0, see http://creativecommons.org/licenses/by/2.0/.
2. Reports of medical cases. *The Oxford Dictionary of Medical Quotations*. Oxford, UK: Oxford University Press.

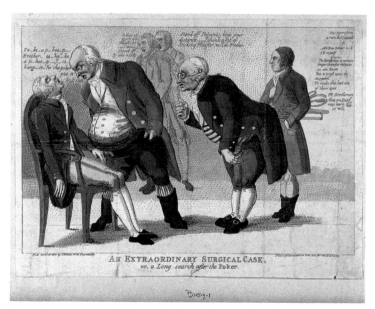

A gagging man surrounded by confused consultants and medical students.
Coloured etching, 1800. Published: S.W. Fores, [London] (50 Piccadilly):
18 April 1800. (Credit: Wellcome Library [1].)

53 A GAGGING MAN SURROUNDED BY CONFUSED CONSULTANTS AND MEDICAL STUDENTS

The role of patients in medical education has evolved over the centuries. In the past, patients were largely helpful if silent props in the process of education - and largely there to be practiced on. At its worst, this meant that patients became depersonalised and were not treated as human beings. Ian Guy captured this attitude well: 'I have yet to see the solitary spleen in bed 5, or the hip replacement on ward 10; visions of a lonesome organ or a prosthesis abound, but do not materialise' (2).

As medical education became more patient-centred, others worried that the pendulum might have swung too far in the opposite direction and that we might be in danger of producing empathetic incompetents. Is there a middle way? According to Raanan Gillon, 'being pleasant, warm, concerned, and, where appropriate, compassionate on the one hand and being medically and scientifically competent on the other are not mutually exclusive attributes' (3).

It is worth wondering how patient-centred these nineteenth-century teachers and learners were. The students in the background are horrified – but not by the plight of the patient. The caption beside them reads: 'Is that all we are to be taught for our money?'

Notes

1. Copyrighted work available under Creative Commons Attribution only licence CC BY 2.0, see http://creativecommons.org/licenses/by/2.0.

2. Guy I. Curious and curiouser? *BMJ* (Published 17 June 2003).

3. Gillon R. Doctors and patients. *BMJ* 1986;292:466.

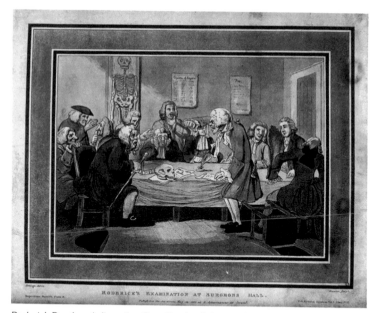

Roderick Random (a licentiate from Scotland) facing a board of medical examiners at Surgeons Hall. Coloured aquatint by J. Stadler, 1800, after S. Collings after T. Smollett. 1800. Published: R. Ackermanns, London. (Credit: Wellcome Library [1].)

54 RODERICK RANDOM (A LICENTIATE FROM SCOTLAND) FACING A BOARD OF MEDICAL EXAMINERS AT SURGEONS' HALL

Roderick Random is a fictional character created by Tobias Smollett, a Scottish poet and novelist. *The Adventures of Roderick Random* (1748) describes the eponymous hero's experiences as an apprentice doctor. He planned to join the navy as a surgeon but first had to go before a board of medical examiners at Surgeons' Hall. He faced a series of questions but the examiners couldn't agree on the answers and so he was asked to leave the room. He passed the exam.

One is reminded of John Rowan Wilson writing about the Royal College of Surgeons. According to Wilson, fellowship at the college 'is decided by examination, and theoretically all Fellows are equal just as theoretically all officers are gentlemen'(2).

The examination in the picture is certainly chaotic: one examiner is standing up, another gesticulating, yet another holds his head in his hands – they are doing almost everything apart from examining. However this is just one of the many adventures that Roderick experiences. The novel is a satire on the hypocrisy and corruption in the medical profession as well as the military and the clergy.

Notes

1. Copyrighted work available under Creative Commons Attribution only licence CC BY 2.0, see http://creativecommons.org/licenses/by/2.0/.
2. Richards P, Stockill S, Foster R, Ingall E. *Learning Medicine*, 17th edn. Cambridge, UK: Cambridge University Press; 2006.

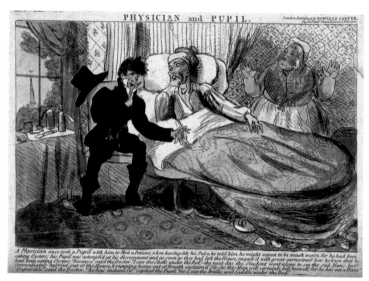

An inexperienced student doctor taking the pulse of a patient in his bed. Coloured etching by A.M. Mills, 1806. Published: Bowles & Carver, London (69 St Paul's Church Yard): 3 February 1806. (Credit: Wellcome Library [1].)

55 AN INEXPERIENCED STUDENT DOCTOR TAKING THE PULSE OF A PATIENT IN HIS BED

Medical students have always learned at the bedside and always will. The question is how to ensure that they learn from experience, with the correct amount of supervision and without harming patients or themselves. Baron Guillaume Dupuytren advised to 'read little, see much, do much' (attributed), but William Stewart Halsted wrote that 'the intern suffers not only from inexperience, but also from over-experience' (2). Each generation of teachers and learners must decide where the balance lies.

In this image, it is worth reflecting on the experience of this medical student and on his learning. The caption underneath reveals what was once a constant of medical education – the narrative or story or joke. Often medical students or patients were the butt of the joke, or sometimes of the apocryphal story. The purpose of the story was usually to make a clinical point, but often said more about the culture of medicine and medical education at the time. Typical characters in such stories were the ignorant patient, the naïve medical student and the wise physician.

Stories, narratives and even jokes can still have an important role in medical education; however, as a profession we might do best to take a wry look at ourselves.

Notes

1. Copyrighted work available under Creative Commons Attribution only licence CC BY 4.0, http://creativecommons.org/licenses/by/4.0/.
2. Halsted WS. The training of the surgeon. *Bull Johns Hopkins Hosp* 1904;15:267.

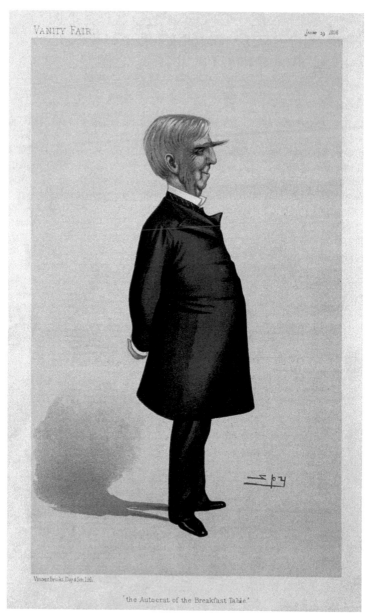

Oliver Wendell Holmes. Coloured lithograph by Sir Leslie Matthew Ward [Spy], 1886. (Credit: Wellcome Library [1].)

56 OLIVER WENDELL HOLMES

Oliver Wendell Holmes, Sr (1809–1894) was an American polymath. He was a renowned physician, educator and author. He coined the term 'Boston Brahmin' to describe those of the upper castes of Boston society – from which he himself had originated. A dedicated reformer, he sometimes became frustrated by the slow pace of change in medicine – once famously saying 'it is so hard to get anything out of the dead hand of medical tradition!' (2). However, Holmes undoubtedly tried. He attempted to admit female students to Harvard Medical School – but both students and faculty resisted. He tried to admit black students to the school but this initiative also foundered. He caused controversy by claiming that doctors were carrying puerperal fever from patient to patient by failing to ensure that they and their instruments were clean.

This lithograph shows Holmes as *The Autocrat of the Breakfast Table* – this was the title of a collection of his essays. The creator of the lithograph was Leslie Matthew Ward – a noted artist and caricaturist. He worked under the pseudonym 'Spy', and the caricatures are sometimes called 'spy cartoons'. His caricatures followed a pattern and this one is no exception: the head and trunk are oversized and somehow held up by miniature legs and feet. However, the caricature is a relatively kind one – the massive eyebrows and sideburns give an impression of gentle academic eccentricity. Holmes' students called him Uncle Oliver.

Notes

1. Copyrighted work available under Creative Commons Attribution only licence CC BY 2.0, see http://creativecommons.org/licenses/by/2.0/.
2. Oliver Wendell Holmes. Medical Essays, *Currents and Counter-Currents in Medical Science*. 1861. Ticknor and Fields, Boston.

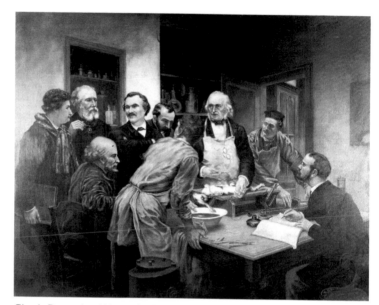

Claude Bernard and his pupils. Oil painting after Léon-Augustin Lhermitte. 1889.
(Credit: Wellcome Library [1].)

57 CLAUDE BERNARD AND HIS PUPILS

Claude Bernard (1813–1878) was a French physiologist and scientist. He became famous for describing homeostasis but as importantly he was among the first to promote the experimental method. He felt that the reality of what we can observe through experiment should be assigned more weight than what ancient scholars might have written: 'When we meet a fact which contradicts a prevailing theory, we must accept the fact and abandon the theory, even when the theory is supported by great names and generally accepted' (2).

Bernard described learning and science as follows: 'Ardent desire for knowledge, in fact, is the one motive attracting and supporting investigators in their efforts; and just this knowledge, really grasped and yet always flying before them, becomes at once their sole torment and their sole happiness' (2). Certainly, an 'ardent desire for knowledge' remains an essential aspiration amongst all students of medicine – of all ages.

Once again this image is most memorable for the interaction between teacher and learner and between learners themselves. The learners are observing, taking notes, leaning forward to get a better view; one seems to be smiling with recognition at the findings. The painting is by Léon Augustin Lhermitte, a French realist painter.

Notes

1. Copyrighted work available under Creative Commons Attribution only licence CC BY 2.0, see http://creativecommons.org/licenses/by/2.0/.
2. Claude Bernard. An Introduction to the Study of Experimental Medicine, Paris, 1865.

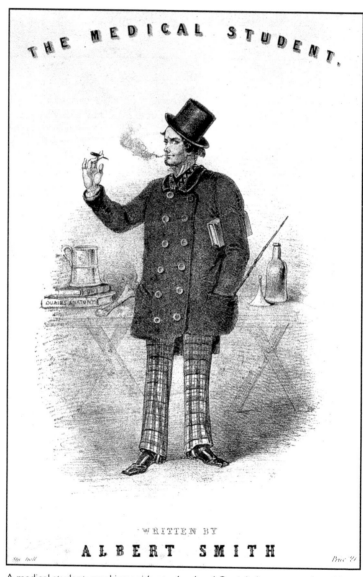

A medical student, smoking, with a tankard and *Quain's Anatomy* on the table. Lithograph, nineteenth century. From: The medical student (song). By: Albert Smith. Published: Brewer and Co./Leoni Lee London. (Credit: Wellcome Library [1].)

58 A MEDICAL STUDENT, SMOKING, WITH A TANKARD AND *QUAIN'S ANATOMY* ON THE TABLE

What are we to make of medical students who smoke cigarettes and drink too much? Here is Keith Ball encouraging an evidence-based and workforce economics approach: 'Medical schools will produce more doctors who will survive to practise medicine till retirement age if their graduates do not smoke cigarettes' (2). And here is Charles Dickens putting it more colourfully: 'a parcel of lazy, idle fellars, that are always smoking and drinking and lounging...a parcel of young cutters and carvers of live people's bodies, that disgraces the lodgings' (3).

In the past, medical schools have often been indulgent of their students who drink and smoke – treating them as prodigal sons who will return to the professional fold on qualifying. However, an inconvenient truth is that physicians have a higher rate of alcohol dependency disorder than that found in the general population. This has led many to rethink professional attitudes to undergraduate behaviour and to the culture of medical schools.

A close examination of the lithograph shows a collection of bottles, bones and books in the background. Also visible is *Quain's Anatomy*. Written by Jones Quain, this was one of the principal anatomical textbooks of its day. It was not intended to serve as a beer mat for students' tankards – as it is in this lithograph.

Notes

1. Copyrighted work available under Creative Commons Attribution only licence CC BY 2.0, see http://creativecommons.org/licenses/by/2.0.
2. Ball K. Medical students and smoking. *BMJ* 1970;4:367.
3. Charles Dickens. *The Pickwick Papers*. 1837. Chapman and Hall. London.

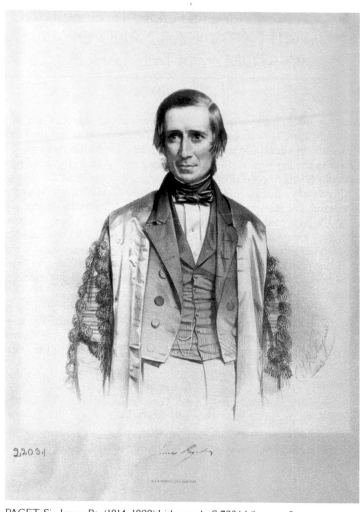

PAGET, Sir James Bt. {1814–1899} Lithograph: S 7906 Library reference no.:
Burgess, Portraits 2203.1. (Credit: Wellcome Library [1].)

59 JAMES PAGET

James Paget (1814–1899) was an English surgeon and pathologist. He described osteitis deformans (Paget's disease of the bone) and intraductal breast cancer (Paget's disease of the nipple). Paget's rise through the ranks of medicine was slow yet inexorable. He shone as an undergraduate – winning prizes and even discovering novel pathogens (such as *Trichinella spiralis*, the cause of trichinosis). On qualifying however he was too poor to afford to become a house surgeon or dresser and eked out a living by writing articles for journals and curating material at the museum of the Royal College of Surgeons.

Continuous study and work from then on were to lead to professorships, lectureships and eventually to his appointment as surgeon extraordinary to Queen Victoria. He became vice chancellor of the University of London in 1883 and remained committed to teaching and learning all his life: 'A very wise old man said that, it would be well if the youngest amongst us would remember that he is not infallible' (2).

This half-length portrait of the robed Paget is by Thomas Herbert Maguire – a well-known artist and lithographer. Academics wearing robes dates back to the Middle Ages when universities were places of religion as well as scholarship.

Notes

1. Copyrighted work available under Creative Commons Attribution only licence CC BY 2.0, see http://creativecommons.org/licenses/by/2.0/.
2. Paget J. An address on the collective investigation of disease. *BMJ* 1883;1:144.

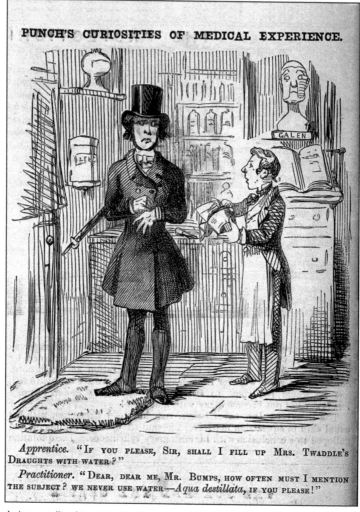

A doctor telling his apprentice how to use language correctly. Wood engraving after J. Leech. 1817–1864. (Credit: Wellcome Library [1].)

60 A DOCTOR TELLING HIS APPRENTICE HOW TO USE LANGUAGE CORRECTLY

This engraving purports to show a doctor telling his apprentice how to use language correctly. However, a close inspection of the narrative shows that the education is more likely to fit the needs of the doctor than the patient. The apprentice asks, 'If you please, Sir, shall I fill up Mrs. Twaddle's draughts with water?' The practitioner replies, 'Dear, dear me, Mr. Bumps, how often must I mention the subject? We never use water – *Aqua destillata*, if you please!' Such behaviour would eventually prompt this reprimand from George Bernard Shaw: 'All professions are a conspiracy against the laity' (2).

The practitioner is likely to be a poor role model for his apprentice, and recent research in medical education has revealed the importance of role models and the effect that they have on learners. The formal outcomes laid out in the curriculum may suggest certain behaviours; however, if the direct supervisors of the learners behave in different ways, then it is likely that the learners will follow the role models. This is true even if the role models demonstrate unprofessional behaviours.

The engraving is by John Leech, an English caricaturist. Leech initially studied to become a doctor at St Bartholomew's Hospital but then abandoned his studies to become an artist.

Notes

1. Copyrighted work available under Creative Commons Attribution only licence CC BY 2.0, see http://creativecommons.org/licenses/by/2.0/.
2. Smith R. Profile of the GMC: The day of judgment comes closer. *BMJ* 1989;298:1241.

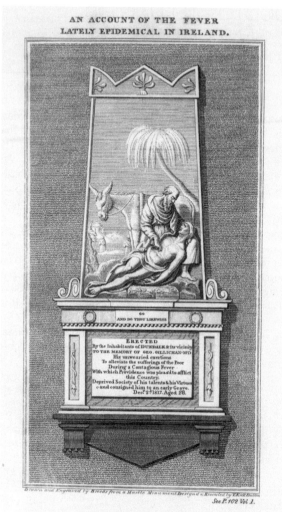

Memorial, erected by the inhabitants of Dundalk in Ireland, to Geo Gillichan, M.D., for his work during the Irish fever epidemic. He died in 1817. From: An account of the rise, progress, and decline of the fever lately epidemical in Ireland, together with communications from physicians in the provinces. And various official documents/By: Francis Barker Published: Baldwin, Cradock and Joy, Dublin: 1821. (Credit: Wellcome Library [1].)

61 MEMORIAL TO A DOCTOR FOR WORK DURING THE IRISH FEVER EPIDEMIC

This memorial was 'erected by the inhabitants of Dundalk in Ireland to Geo Gillichan, M.D., for his work during the Irish fever epidemic. He died in 1817' (2). During fever epidemics of the past, physicians would sometimes refuse to see patients out of fear that they would contract the fever themselves. The Irish fever epidemic was caused by typhus; it affected the poorest sections of society as well as those who came in close contact with them – primarily physicians and the clergy. So physicians who worried about contracting the disease themselves had considerable justification for their worry. However, Geo Gillichan was clearly an honourable exception. As James Black wrote 'but the profession must not complain, for "Salus populi suprema lex"' (The welfare of the people shall be the supreme law.) (3).

The memorial depicts a traveller helping an ill man by the roadside – possibly an allusion to the Good Samaritan. The image was taken from the book *An Account of the Rise, Progress, and Decline of the Fever Lately Epidemical in Ireland, Together with Communications from Physicians in the Provinces* by Francis Barker and John Cheyne. Francis Barker physician and founder of the first Irish fever hospital.

Notes

1. Copyrighted work available under Creative Commons Attribution only licence CC BY 2.0, see http://creativecommons.org/licenses/by/2.0/.
2. http://wellcomeimages.org/ (accessed 9 March 2016).
3. Black J. Dr. Black on medical reform. *Prov Med Surg J* 1840;1(9):147.

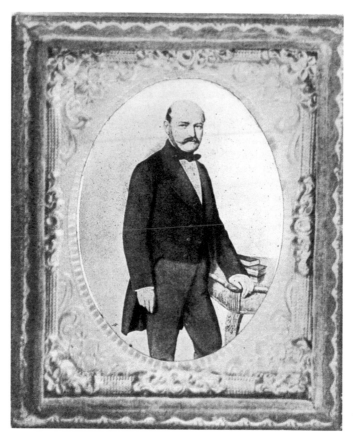

Ignaz Philipp Semmelweis. (Credit: Wellcome Library [1].)

62 IGNAZ PHILIPP SEMMELWEIS

Ignaz Philipp Semmelweis (1818–1865) was a Hungarian physician. He discovered that simple antiseptic procedures (such as handwashing) could markedly reduce the occurrence of puerperal fever and save mothers' lives. Semmelweis worked at two obstetric clinics and found that they had markedly different maternal mortality rates. He studied both clinics to discover what could account for the difference; however, the only thing he could find was that one of the clinics was for trainee midwives and the other for medical students. Then a friend of Semmelweis, Jakob Kolletschka, died of sepsis after being cut by a medical student's scalpel during an autopsy. Semmelweis quickly made the link – medical students were infecting pregnant women with material from the autopsies (midwives did not attend autopsies). He introduced strict handwashing, and mortality rates fell dramatically.

However his findings were rejected by the medical establishment. He complained that 'most medical lecture halls continue to resound with lectures on epidemic childbed fever and with discourses against my theories' (2). His protests against the medical establishment grew increasingly angry and he was eventually committed to an asylum. He died of blood poisoning in 1865 – possibly caused by wounds inflicted by a beating from the asylum guards.

Notes

1. Copyrighted work available under Creative Commons Attribution only licence CC BY 2.0, see http://creativecommons.org/licenses/by/2.0/.
2. Semmelweis I, Carter KC. *Etiology, Concept and Prophylaxis of Childbed Fever*. Madison, WI: University of Wisconsin Press; 1983/[1861].

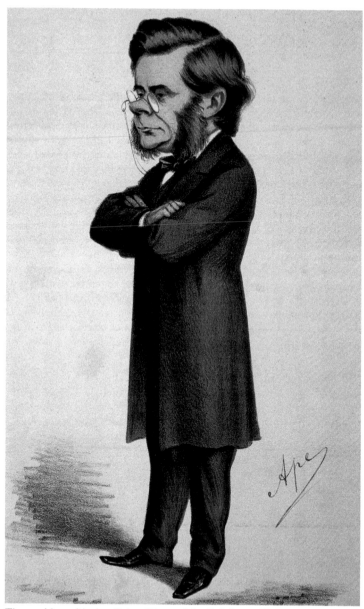

Thomas Henry Huxley. Colour lithograph by C. Pellegrini [Ape], 1871.
(Credit: Wellcome Library [1].)

63 THOMAS HENRY HUXLEY

Thomas Henry Huxley (1825–1895) was an anatomist and a supporter of Darwin's theory of evolution. He had a strong influence on the modernisation of medical curricula in the nineteenth century. He was one of the first medical teachers to realise the importance of medical students learning how to learn: '…and I am quite sure a very considerable number of young men spend a large portion of their first session simply learning how to learn in a fashion that is entirely new to them' (2). Huxley was also forthright about what he saw as the primary purpose of education: 'Perhaps the most valuable result of all education is the ability to make yourself do the thing you have to do, when it ought to be done, whether you like it or not' (3). Huxley's knowledge, teaching skills and values were to attract students of the highest calibre. His students included William Rutherford, E. Ray Lankester, Michael Foster and William Flower.

Huxley was nicknamed Darwin's bulldog for his aggressive defence of Darwin's ideas, and this cartoon shows the 'bulldog' in a typically forthright and aggressive pose. The caricaturist was Carlo Pellegrini, nicknamed Ape, who worked for *Vanity Fair*.

Notes

1. Copyrighted work available under Creative Commons Attribution only licence CC BY 2.0, see http://creativecommons.org/licenses/by/2.0.
2. Huxley T. Introductory address on the intervention of the state in the affairs of the medical profession. *BMJ* 1883;2:709.
3. http://thinkexist.com/quotes/thomas_henry_huxley/3.html (accessed 4 April 2015).

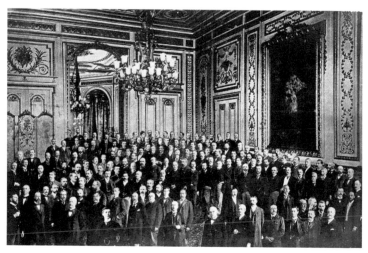

Lord Lister with his house surgeons and dressers, 1861–1893. (Credit: Wellcome Library [1].)

64 JOSEPH LISTER WITH HIS HOUSE SURGEONS AND DRESSERS

Joseph Lister (1827–1912) was an English surgeon who introduced antiseptic surgery to the United Kingdom. Building on the ideas of Louis Pasteur, he used carbolic acid to clean surgical wounds. He also insisted that his surgical team use aseptic technique when operating. Carbolic acid was applied by spraying – prompting one onlooker to intone 'Let us spray' when the solemn Lister entered the operating room 'followed in procession by his train of dressers' (2). However Lister's studies showed that using antiseptics, washing hands and wearing gloves drastically reduced the incidence of surgical site infections. Semmelweis had shown largely the same outcomes many years before, but Lister's championing of these ideas meant that they became accepted.

Here is Lister summarising the conclusions of his research: 'But since the antiseptic treatment has been brought into full operation, and wounds and abscesses no longer poison the atmosphere with putrid exhalations, my wards, though in other respects under precisely the same circumstances as before, have completely changed their character; so that during the last nine months not a single instance of pyaemia, hospital gangrene, or erysipelas has occurred in them' (3).

Famously Lister came out of retirement in 1902 to advise on the management of Edward VII's appendicitis. Lister offered advice on antisepsis in surgery and the king survived.

Here is Lister with his house surgeons and dressers. I can definitely count over 150: could this be a record?

Notes

1. Copyrighted work available under Creative Commons Attribution only licence CC BY 2.0, see http://creativecommons.org/licenses/by/2.0/.

2. Granshaw I. Upon this principle I have based a practice. In Pickstone JV (Ed.), *Medical Innovations in Historical Perspective*. New York: St Martin's Press; 1992.

3. http://www.gutenberg.org/cache/epub/5694/pg5694.html (accessed 18 April 2015).

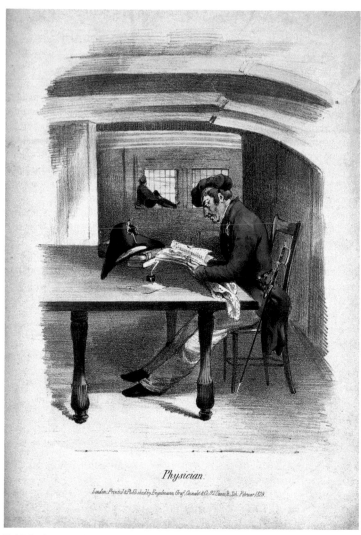

Published: printed and published by Engelmann, Graf, Coindet & Co, London (92 Dean St Soho): February 1829. (Credit: Wellcome Library [1].)

65 A NAVAL PHYSICIAN IN UNIFORM STUDYING BOOKS AT A LARGE TABLE

> If we take into account the pivotal role that reading has in a doctor's continuous learning then reading should be generously honoured, allowing doctors to meet at least half of any set annual standard of credit points by reporting their reading and its perceived influence on their practice.
>
> **Hans Asbjørn Holm (2)**

Reading has always been a core part of medical education but has not always received the attention and credit it deserves. Do we do enough in medical schools to engender effective study habits and lifelong reading skills? It is probable that we could never do enough.

Certainly, there is a massive amount of new medical knowledge that is published every year and it is impossible for a single individual to read all of it, never mind learn it. Thus, the modern emphasis in continuous professional development has turned to critical reading skills, whereby physicians consider the validity and relevance of the content that they read and reflect on how they might apply it in practice.

This naval physician strikes a concentrated pose – but what of his surroundings? Who is the figure in the windowsill? Is this nineteenth-century distance learning? This would be more likely if he were aboard a ship but the environment doesn't suggest this.

Notes

1. Copyrighted work available under Creative Commons Attribution only licence CC BY 2.0, see http://creativecommons.org/licenses/by/2.0/.
2. Holm HA. Should doctors get CME points for reading? Yes: Relaxing documentation doesn't imply relaxing accountability. *BMJ* 2000;320:394.

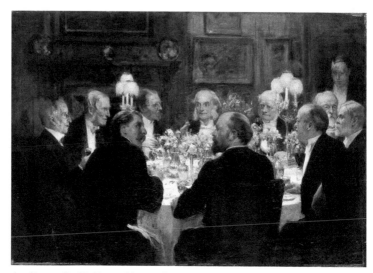

An Octave for Mr Ernest Hart at Sir Henry Thompson's house. Oil painting by
Solomon Joseph Solomon R.A., ca. 1897. (Credit: Wellcome Library [1].)

66 AN OCTAVE FOR MR ERNEST HART

Ernest Hart (1835–1898) was a surgeon, educator and editor of the *BMJ*. He started his studies at St George's Hospital and worked as an eye surgeon at St Mary's Hospital, eventually progressing to become dean. He worked at *the Lancet* and was appointed editor of the *BMJ* in 1866. He transformed the *BMJ* from a provincial journal into a respected national publication. Hart was a campaigning editor and championed a number of causes including military medicine, medical education for women, public health, infectious disease prevention and vaccination. He was a stout defender of the journal and editorial freedom: 'Editors must have enemies. Woe to the journalist of whom only good is said' (2). According the *Journal of the American Medical Association*, as a writer Hart 'was forceful, accurate and aggressive. As a man he was unassuming, polite and agreeable. As a physician he was well informed and in certain lines in advance of his time' (3).

This picture is intriguingly titled An Octave for Mr Ernest Hart. Octaves were dinner parties hosted by the surgeon Professor Henry Thompson. Eight courses and eight wines were served to eight guests. Why then are 10 people seated? The other two were the host and the guest of honour – in this case Ernest Hart. The painting is by Solomon Joseph Solomon, an English artist and member of the Royal Academy.

Notes

1. Copyrighted work available under Creative Commons Attribution only licence CC BY 2.0, see http://creativecommons.org/licenses/by/2.0/.
2. Jewell D. So then, farewell: An editor writes. *Br J Gen Pract* 2009;59(569):952–953.
3. http://jama.jamanetwork.com/article.aspx?articleid=464483 (accessed 8 April 2015).

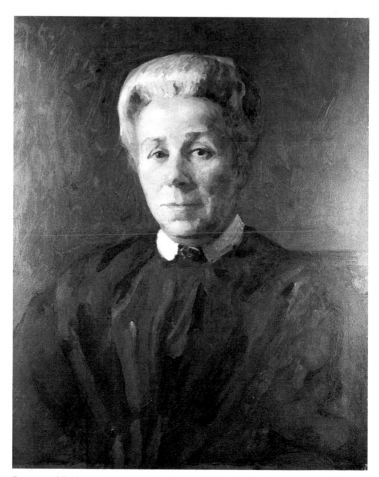

Portrait of E. Garrett Anderson, half-length. (Credit: Wellcome Library [1].)

67 ELIZABETH GARRETT ANDERSON

Elizabeth Garrett Anderson (1836–1917) was the first woman in Britain to gain a medical licence. She did so in 1865 after a long battle with the medical authorities. Within 10 years, she was to found the first school of medicine for women in the United Kingdom. By 1895, she was able to say, 'the medical education for women is now so far organised in England that there is very little to say about it. It is almost as easy at this moment for a woman to get a complete medical education in England, Scotland, or Ireland, as it is for a man' (2).

Elizabeth Garrett was born in 1836 in Whitechapel, East London. She received her education first from her mother, then from a governess and then finally at a private boarding school. She worked initially as a nurse and tried to enrol in medical school. On being refused, she employed a private tutor. She eventually received a certificate in anatomy and physiology and a licence to practise medicine from the Society of Apothecaries. After qualifying, she couldn't get a post in a hospital and so set up her own practice in London. She got married and had children but did not give up her medical practice. She claimed that 'a doctor leads two lives, the professional and the private, and the boundaries between the two are never traversed' (3).

Notes

1. Copyrighted work available under Creative Commons Attribution only licence CC BY 2.0, see http://creativecommons.org/licenses/by/2.0/.
2. Anderson EG. Medical Education of Women: The Qualification of Female Practitioners. *BMJ* 1895;2:608.
3. Manton J. *Elizabeth Garrett Anderson*. Methuen; 1965, p. 261.

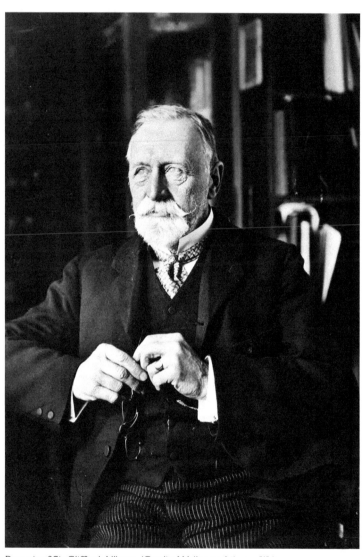

Portrait of Sir Clifford Allbutt. (Credit: Wellcome Library [1].)

68 THOMAS CLIFFORD ALLBUTT

Thomas Clifford Allbutt (1836–1925) was an English physician and inventor of the pocket thermometer. Before his invention, thermometers were about a foot long and patients needed to hold them for 20 minutes. Allbutt also introduced ophthalmoscopy and microscopy to the hospitals where he worked. His manuscript *On the Use of the Ophthalmoscope in Diseases of the Nervous System and of the Kidneys* described the usefulness of ophthalmoscopy in the diagnosis of neurological and psychiatric diseases. His book *System of Medicine* was widely hailed as the definitive textbook of the era.

Allbutt was an early advocate of curriculum reform and rationalisation: 'for two generations we have been loading and loading this brief curriculum as if we desired to teach many things ill rather than a few things well' (2). On his death, the medical correspondent of *The Times* wrote that Allbutt 'urged continually on his students the value of clear thinking and cultivated expression; and his own writings bore witness in every line to the store which he set on that proper equipment of character, disciplined emotion and imagination fitted with exact knowledge' (3).

Notes

1. Copyrighted work available under Creative Commons Attribution only licence CC BY 2.0, see http://creativecommons.org/licenses/by/2.0/.

2. Allbutt TC. An address on medical education in London: Delivered at King's College Hospital on October 3rd, 1905, at the Opening of the Medical Session. *BMJ* 1905;2:913.

3. http://en.wikisource.org/wiki/The_Times/1925/Obituary/Thomas_Clifford_Allbutt (accessed 8 April 2015).

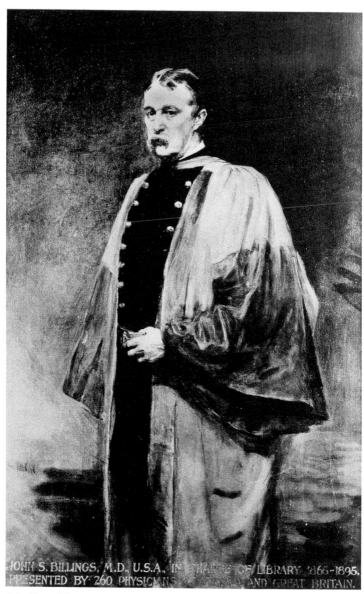

JOHN S. BILLINGS, M.D., U.S.A., IN CHARGE OF LIBRARY 1865-1895.
PRESENTED BY 260 PHYSICIANS OF AMERICA AND GREAT BRITAIN.

John Shaw Billings. Oil painting. (Credit: Wellcome Library [1].)

69 JOHN SHAW BILLINGS

John Shaw Billings (1838–1913) was an American surgeon. He developed the Library of the Surgeon General's Office in the United States which was to become the National Library of Medicine. He was one of the first to realise the importance of high-quality medical informatics in the delivery of both medical education and clinical care. Billings was responsible for setting up Index Medicus, a comprehensive index of articles in medical journals. Today, the National Library of Medicine is the biggest medical library in the world. It contains more than seven million journals, books, manuscripts and images.

Billings was also a strong believer in the importance of ongoing medical education following qualification: 'The education of the doctor which goes on after he has his degree is, after all, the most important part of his education' (2). Today, there is growing interest in how the discipline of medical informatics and medical education can be integrated. This would enable faster translation of research into practice and medical education that is more closely linked to the needs of the physician.

In this photograph, Billings is wearing academic robes and underneath what appears to be a military uniform – he was a medical inspector in the army during the civil war.

Notes

1. Copyrighted work available under Creative Commons Attribution only licence CC BY 2.0, see http://creativecommons.org/licenses/by/2.0.
2. *Boston Medical and Surgical Journal*, 1894;131:140.

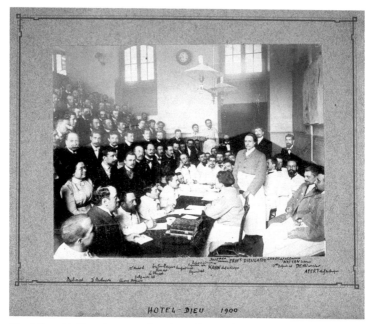

Dieulafoy with his assistants and students during a lecture at l'Hôtel-Dieu.
Photograph, 1900. (Credit: Wellcome Library [1].)

70 DIEULAFOY WITH HIS ASSISTANTS AND STUDENTS DURING A LECTURE AT THE HÔTEL-DIEU

Paul Georges Dieulafoy (1839–1911) was a French surgeon and teacher. He taught at the Hôtel-Dieu in Paris and conducted research and teaching on the appendix – famously declaring that 'the medical treatment of acute appendicitis does not exist' (2). This statement was true at the time; however, it predated the antibiotic era. He described Dieulafoy's triad – a constellation of signs of acute appendicitis, discovered Dieulafoy's lesion – a rare cause of upper gastrointestinal bleeding and invented Dieulafoy's apparatus – a pump to evacuate pleural effusions.

This photograph shows Dieulafoy at the Hôtel-Dieu – the oldest hospital in Paris. It was founded in 651 by Saint Landry and is still a working hospital today. Its initial mission was to provide care for poor people; today it is a place of clinical care, research and education, and it continues to put the patient at the centre of its activities (one of its goals is to ensure that patients are fully informed of their illnesses).

Dieulafoy is clearly in his pomp in this image – surrounded by assistants and students. The photograph is posed – some are looking at the lecturer, some at the camera. Dieulafoy can at least console himself that no one is looking at the clock – showing that he has probably got 20 minutes to go.

Notes

1. Copyrighted work available under Creative Commons Attribution only licence CC BY 2.0, see http://creativecommons.org/licenses/by/2.0.
2. http://en.wikipedia.org/wiki/Paul_Georges_Dieulafoy (accessed 9 March 2016).

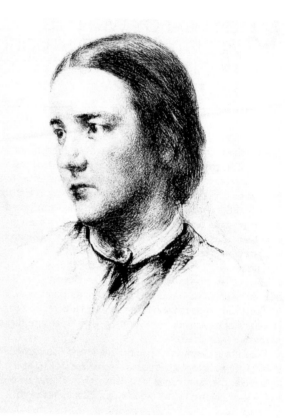

Head and shoulders portrait of Sophia Jex-Blake. (Credit: Wellcome Library [I].)

71 SOPHIA JEX-BLAKE

Sophia Jex-Blake (1840–1912) was an English physician and teacher. She was one of the first women to qualify in medicine in the United Kingdom. After a long struggle, she eventually convinced Edinburgh Medical School to accept her as a student. There she attended segregated lectures with six other women. Unfortunately she failed her exams in Edinburgh but continued to study and eventually obtained a medical degree from the University of Berne. Soon afterwards, she became registered with the General Medical Council. After qualifying, she went on to help found two medical schools for women – in London and in Edinburgh. She also set up a hospital for women in Edinburgh – she broadly thought that the role of female doctors was to care for women.

She promoted good learning habits amongst medical students of both sexes: she encouraged students to learn steadily, to be patient and to only take on what they can achieve. According to Jex-Blake 'girls as well as boys often break down quite unnecessarily, not because their health is defective, but because they study in a foolish and headstrong way, ignoring the ordinary laws of hygiene, and destroying their own future by attempting the impossible in the present' (2).

Notes

1. Copyrighted work available under Creative Commons Attribution only licence CC BY 2.0, see http://creativecommons.org/licenses/by/.
2. Jex-Blake S. Medical education of women. *BMJ* 1895;2:869.

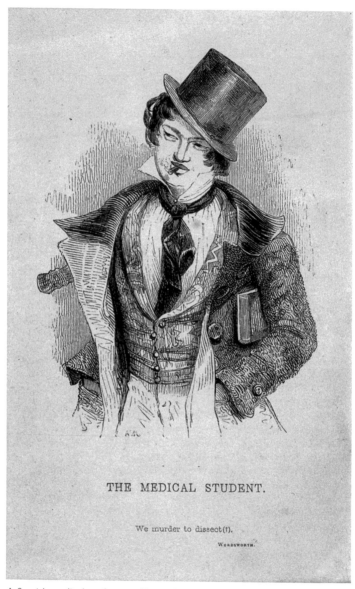

THE MEDICAL STUDENT.

We murder to dissect(†).

WORDSWORTH.

A foppish medical student smoking a cigarette – denoting a cavalier attitude. 1840.
By: Joseph Kenny Meadows after: William Wordsworth and John Orrin Smith.
(Credit: Wellcome Library [1].)

72 A FOPPISH MEDICAL STUDENT SMOKING A CIGARETTE, DENOTING A CAVALIER ATTITUDE

What should we expect of medical students? Should we expect them to adhere to high standards of ethical and professional behaviours at all times? Or is that expecting too much? There are two schools of thought. Some are concerned that moral development may regress during medical school. For example Shimon Glick has written that 'unfortunately there are troubling, if inconclusive, data that suggest that during medical school the ethical behaviour of medical students does not necessarily improve; indeed, moral development may actually stop or even regress' (2). On the other hand, some think that medical students should be allowed a wide berth. Roger Allen has put it colourfully: 'we need reprobates, beer spillers, card sharps, bong puffers, the irreverent and the like in medical students. It is their job' (3).

At the core of the debate is the extent to which behaviour at medical school predicts behaviour after graduation. Many students mature significantly upon graduation and put their student days behind them. However, there is some evidence that doctors who run into trouble with the regulatory authorities had often showed warning signs of this while still at medical school.

Certainly this medical student doesn't fill you with confidence. Everything about him seems lopsided – his hat, his cigarette and possibly his ethical values.

Notes

1. Copyrighted work available under Creative Commons Attribution only licence CC BY 2.0, see http://creativecommons.org/licenses/by/2.0.
2. Glick SM. Cheating at medical school: Schools need a culture that simply makes dishonest behaviour unacceptable. *BMJ* 2001;322:250.
3. Allen RKA. Bring me your reprobates. *BMJ* (Published 12 May 2010).

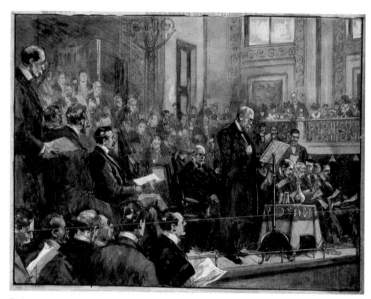

Robert Koch reading his address to a conference at St James's Hall, Piccadilly. Gouache by F.C. Dickinson, 1901. (Credit: Wellcome Library [1].)

73 ROBERT KOCH READING HIS ADDRESS TO A CONFERENCE AT ST JAMES

Robert Koch (1843–1910) was a German microbiologist and scientist. He isolated the microorganisms that cause anthrax, tuberculosis and cholera. He set out four postulates on the causation of infectious disease, which remain the gold standard for the detection of the cause of any disease. His ground-breaking research attracted students from around the world who came to his centres to learn. He was keen to share his discoveries with the world and share credit with his co-researchers. One of his assistants was called Petri.

Koch remained a modest man to the end of his life despite his many achievements. 'If my efforts have led to greater success than usual, this is due, I believe, to the fact that during my wanderings in the field of medicine, I have strayed onto paths where the gold was still lying by the wayside. It takes a little luck to be able to distinguish gold from dross, but that is all' (2).

Here is Koch addressing a conference at St James's Hall. He is well prepared; he has a stand, lecture notes, even drinking water, but does he have his audience's attention?

Notes

1. Copyrighted work available under Creative Commons Attribution only licence CC BY 2.0, see http://creativecommons.org/licenses/by/2.0/.
2. 'Robert Koch', *Journal of Outdoor Life* 1908;5:164–169.

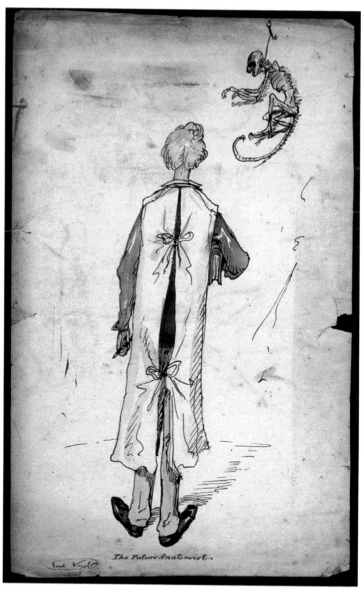

The Future Anatomist

A posterior view of a medical student with a surgical gown untidily tied up.
Coloured pen drawing by E. Griset. (1844–1907). (Credit: Wellcome Library [1].)

74 A POSTERIOR VIEW OF A MEDICAL STUDENT WITH A SURGICAL GOWN UNTIDILY TIED UP

For every medical student that smokes and 'disgraces the lodgings', there is the conscientious student who is hesitant, uncertain, eager to learn – the educational equivalent of the worried well. This rather bookish student seems to embody hesitancy as he approaches his future anatomical studies. Or perhaps he is worried by the amount that he feels he will have to learn.

Henry Souttar wrote in 1938 that 'the medical curriculum has reached the limit of human endurance, and it is only the genius of the medical student for clearing his brain completely after every examination that enables him to preserve his sanity' (2). Souttar's statement rings true and says much about how curricula were created and how medical students were expected to learn. Clearly the content of the curriculum was only there to help students pass examinations and was to be forgotten about immediately afterwards. Modern medical curricula should encourage healthier and more practical study skills. The curriculum should be closely linked to practice so that learning for the long term will be necessary. More thought should also be given to the learner's emotional state – curricula should help develop well-balanced learners who in turn will become well-balanced practitioners.

Notes

1. Copyrighted work available under Creative Commons Attribution only licence CC BY 4.0, http://creativecommons.org/licenses/by/4.0.
2. Langdon-Brown W. The medical curriculum and present-day needs. *BMJ* 1938;2:481.

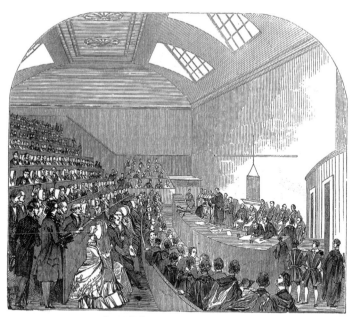

"CAPPING" OF DOCTORS OF MEDICINE, AT EDINBURGH.

Doctors receiving their degrees in a degree ceremony, Edinburgh. Published: Illustrated London News, London, 1845. (Credit: Wellcome Library [1].)

75 DOCTORS RECEIVING THEIR DEGREES IN A DEGREE CEREMONY, EDINBURGH

> But education does not happen to end with registration, or qualification, with the obtaining of a commission, a diploma, or a degree, and there is no professional life in which this truth can be seen more clearly than in the medical life, in relation to which it is stark staleness to say that education never ceases and that the longer we practise our calling the more we have the opportunity of learning, of testing that learning, and of obtaining its rewards.
>
> ***Samuel Squire Sprigge (2)***

Continuous professional development didn't start in the 1990s – it has always been part of the make-up of professionals. Modern medical education has merely formalised a process that has always taken place. However, medical education concepts can claim to have made a significant contribution to best practice in continuous professional development. As a result doctors are now more likely to do learning based on their learning needs, to learn using a variety of types of resources and to plan how their learning will have an impact on their clinical practice.

Despite more emphasis on continuous professional development, the graduation ceremony remains important. Here we can see the traditional 'capping' ceremony taking place with the new doctor at the front bowing to receive his 'cap'.

Notes

1. Copyrighted work available under Creative Commons Attribution only licence CC BY 4.0, http://creativecommons.org/licenses/by/4.0.
2. Sprigge SS. An address on prizes and performances: Delivered at the Opening of the Medical Session at St George's Hospital, on October 1st. *BMJ* 1910;2:1024.

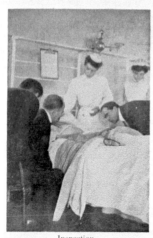

Inspection

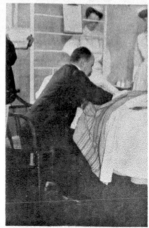

Palpation

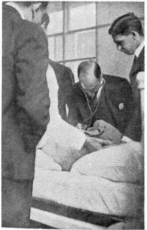

Auscultation

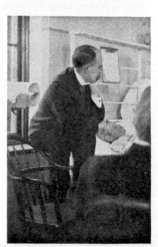

Contemplation

SNAPSHOTS OF OSLER AT THE BEDSIDE

From snapshots taken by T.W.Clarke

William Osler at the bedside of patients. From: The life of Sir William Osler. By: Harvey Cushing Published: Clarendon Press, Oxford, 1925. Volume 1, Facing page 552. (Credit: Wellcome Library [1].)

76 WILLIAM OSLER

William Osler (1849–1919) was one of the founding fathers of Johns Hopkins Hospital. He introduced clinical training at the bedside for medical students and trainee doctors. He also set up residencies for doctors in training. Residents lived in the hospital and learned by delivering hands-on care for patients. He developed the concept of a clinical clerkship for undergraduates, whereby senior medical students spent time on the wards taking histories, conducting examinations and following up patients. He claimed to 'desire no epitaph … than the statement that I taught medical students in the wards, as I regard this as by far the most useful and important work I have been called upon to do' (2).

This image shows Osler in action, demonstrating the skills of inspection, palpation and auscultation. The fourth clinical skill comes last – contemplation. These relatively simple skills would help him discover the following eponymous signs, syndromes and diseases: Osler's nodes, Osler's sign, Osler–Rendu–Weber disease and Osler–Libman–Sacks syndrome.

Remarkably, Osler still found time to discover a fellow educator – Egerton Yorrick Davis. Davis was a retired U.S. Army surgeon who conducted a prolific, if bizarre, correspondence with medical societies until his untimely death in a drowning accident in 1884. It turned out that William Osler invented Davis as a long-standing practical joke against learned societies and even more learned journals.

Notes

1. Copyrighted work available under Creative Commons Attribution only licence CC BY 2.0, see http://creativecommons.org/licenses/by/2.0/.

2. Osler W. *Aequanimitas, With Other Addresses to Medical Students, Nurses and Practitioners of Medicine*, 4th edn. London, UK: The Keynes Press; 1984.

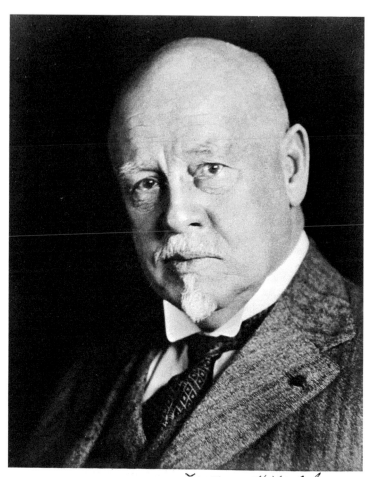

William Henry Welch. Photograph. (Credit: Wellcome Library [I].)

77 WILLIAM HENRY WELCH

William Henry Welch (1850–1934) was an American physician and pathologist. He was one of the founders of Johns Hopkins School of Medicine and subsequently of the Johns Hopkins School of Hygiene and Public Health. Dedicated to medical education, he became known as the 'Dean of American Medicine'. He was another advocate of lifelong learning: 'medical education is not completed at the medical school: it is only begun' (2).

If medical educators were judged by the achievements of their students, then Welch could claim to be one of the foremost – of his own or any time. Walter Reed, George Whipple, Peyton Rous all studied under Welch and were to go on to discover diseases, found institutions and win Nobel prizes. According to one account, his students 'could not fail to appreciate the lucidity of his presentations, the breadth of his knowledge of the subject matter under consideration, nor the faculty, which he possessed to an unusual degree, of investing each topic which he discussed with a measure of interest that seemed almost to transcend, at times, the intrinsic value of the subject itself. Indeed, many a time the discussion which Dr. Welch gave of a colleague's paper in the meetings of the Johns Hopkins Medical Society was a clearer and better exposition of the subject than was the paper itself' (3). Welch himself discovered *Clostridium welchii*, now more commonly known as *Clostridium perfringens*.

Although some figures in the history of medical education were distant from their students, Welch certainly was not. His students called him Popsy.

Notes

1. Copyrighted work available under Creative Commons Attribution only licence CC BY 2.0, see http://creativecommons.org/licenses/by/2.0.
2. *Bulletin of the Harvard Medical School Association* 1892;3:55.
3. Chesney AM. William Henry Welch, a Tribute on the Centenary of his Birth, April 1950. Available at the Alan Mason Chesney Medical Archives of the Johns Hopkins Medical Institutions.

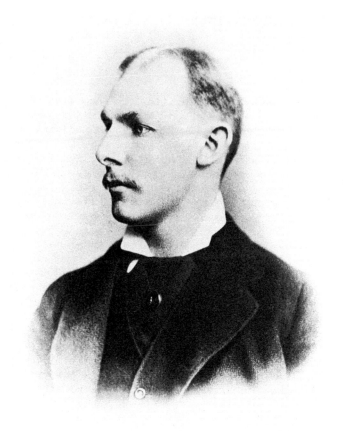

© Jeffres, Baltimore

Portrait of W. S. Halsted, head and shoulders. From: Surgical papers. Published: Johns Hopkins Press, Baltimore: 1924. Volume I. (Credit: Wellcome Library [1].)

78 WILLIAM STEWART HALSTED

William Stewart Halsted (1852–1922) was another founding father of Johns Hopkins Medical School. He set up the first formal training programme in surgery in the United States. This was a competency-based programme where trainee surgeons moved on to the next level of training once Halsted was satisfied with their current competence. According to Cameron, it is Halsted's contribution to medical education that will be his most lasting legacy: 'no matter how great the magnitude of advances by Halsted and his peers during the evolution of the modem era of surgery in this country, without a mechanism for passing them on to others and a mechanism for educating young clinicians-scientists, such as is provided by the Halsted surgical residency training system, their continuation could not be assured, nor their promulgation and extension promoted' (2). Halsted put himself in the place of trainees and developed much insight into the minds of those in training.

Halsted also put himself in the place of the patient – albeit with unfortunate results. He experimented with the use of cocaine as an anaesthetic but ended up addicted to it. In weaning himself off cocaine, he became addicted to morphine. When working at Johns Hopkins, his theatre nurse complained of dermatitis caused by using antiseptic. Halsted was inspired to help design the first set of surgical gloves. The theatre nurse became his wife.

This image is formal and posed, and gives little insight into the powerhouse yet eccentric educator, researcher and clinician that was behind the mask.

Notes

1. Copyrighted work available under Creative Commons Attribution only licence CC BY 2.0, see http://creativecommons.org/licenses/by/2.0.
2. Cameron JL. William Stewart Halsted. Our surgical heritage. *Ann Surg* 1997;225(5):445–458.

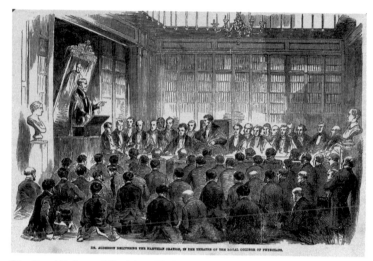

DR. ALDERSON DELIVERING THE HARVEIAN ORATION, IN THE THEATRE OF THE ROYAL COLLEGE OF PHYSICIANS.

The Royal College of Physicians, Trafalgar Square: A meeting of the college for the Harveian lecture. Wood engraving, 1854. Published: London. (Credit: Wellcome Library [1].)

79 THE ROYAL COLLEGE OF PHYSICIANS, TRAFALGAR SQUARE: A MEETING OF THE COLLEGE FOR THE HARVEIAN LECTURE

Educational meetings have always been part of the continuous professional development of doctors. This image, however, is more suggestive of a religious service than a medical meeting. The high priest of medical knowledge appears to be holding forth from his pulpit. His acolytes look upwards in reverential silence.

Modern medical education meetings should be different. Ideally, they should be about the coming together of a faculty of speakers of national or international repute and a cohort of delegates who are eager to learn. Best practice in education leads to an exchange between faculty and learners. Medical education should be more than just knowledge transfer – delegates should be encouraged to learn actively, to ask questions, to discuss with colleagues and to reflect on how their practice might change as a result of their learning. Educational meetings should be more than a simple once-off; learners should plan how their attendance at meetings will help them fulfil their learning needs or learn according to a set curriculum.

Is that all medical meetings should be about? According to Jules Older, they 'should be about learning and change (never mind job seeking, flirtation, tax breaks, drinking, and the rest of the conference's hidden curriculum)' (2). And how often should doctors attend? According to Francis Martin Rouse Walshe, 'symposia, like hard liquor, should be taken in reasonable measure, at appropriate intervals' (3).

Notes

1. Copyrighted work available under Creative Commons Attribution only licence CC BY 2.0, see http://creativecommons.org/licenses/by/2.0.
2. Older J. Personal view. *BMJ* 1985;290:930.
3. Walshe FMR. *Perspect Biol Med* 1959;2:197.

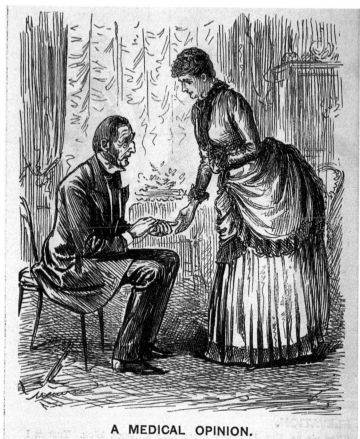

A MEDICAL OPINION.

Eminent Physician. "I FEEL VERY QUEER. I WONDER WHAT CAN BE THE MATTER?"

Anxious Wife. "SHALL I SEND FOR DOCTOR PILCOX OR DOCTOR SQUILLS?"

E. P. "NO, NO."   *A. W.* "OR ANY OTHER DOCTOR?"

E. P. "NO; WE ALL GO IN FOR THINKING EACH OTHER SUCH HUMBUGS!"

An ill physician refusing to let his wife call another doctor. Wood engraving after G. Du Maurier. Published: London. (Credit: Wellcome Library [1].)

80 AN ILL PHYSICIAN REFUSING TO LET HIS WIFE CALL ANOTHER DOCTOR

'I haven't got time to be sick!' he said. 'People need me'. For he was a country doctor, and he did not know what it was to spare himself.

Don Marquis (2)

Why do good doctors make bad patients? There are probably lots of reasons, but being unwilling to spare oneself must be a common cause. Doctors can become ill for a variety of reasons, including both physical and mental ones. Modern professionalism should be about knowing when to stop rather than continuing on and possibly harming patients in the process. And modern medical education should be about helping students learn about illnesses that might affect them and engendering behaviours that will enable them to stop when they are unwell. In this regard, the culture of medicine and medical education must change. The ideal doctor should no longer be a female or male superhero who never shows weakness, but a team player who is mindful of their own well-being as well as that of their patients.

And the reason this physician doesn't want his wife to call another doctor? Because 'we all go in for thinking each other such humbugs!'

Notes

1. Copyrighted work available under Creative Commons Attribution only licence CC BY 2.0, see http://creativecommons.org/licenses/by/2.0.
2. Country Doctor, see https://franciscogarrigamd.wordpress.com/2016/01/23/transitions/ (accessed 9 March 2016).

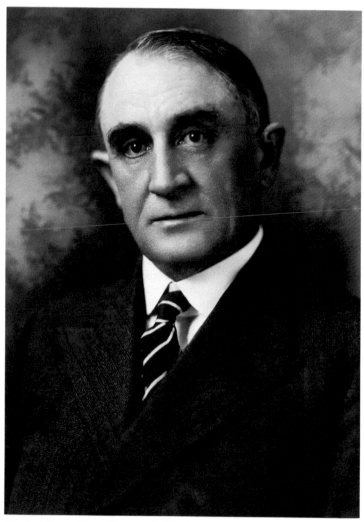

Charles Horace Mayo. Photograph. (Credit: Wellcome Library [1].)

81 CHARLES HORACE MAYO

Charles Horace Mayo (1865–1939) was an American surgeon. Along with his brother William James Mayo, he founded the Mayo Clinic. The Mayo brothers were among the first to develop the concept of medical specialisation: at the Mayo Clinic, doctors worked together in caring for patients with complex medical problems. The clinic's innovative system was to recruit some of the most renowned medical specialists of their day. Charles Mayo's particular specialty was thyroid and cataract surgeries. Mayo was also an early proponent of social accountability in medicine – the clinic treated large numbers of poor patients.

Mayo developed close links with the local medical school and was among the first to recognise the relationship between teaching, learning and patient care. According to Mayo 'the safest thing for a patient is to be in the hands of a man engaged in teaching medicine. In order to be a teacher of medicine the doctor must always be a student' (2). This is a dictum that remains true to this day, and the Mayo Clinic remains an institution that stands for excellence in medicine, medical education and research.

Notes

1. Copyrighted work available under Creative Commons Attribution only licence CC BY 2.0, see http://creativecommons.org/licenses/by/2.0/.
2. *Proceedings of the Staff Meetings of the Mayo Clinic* 1927;2:223.

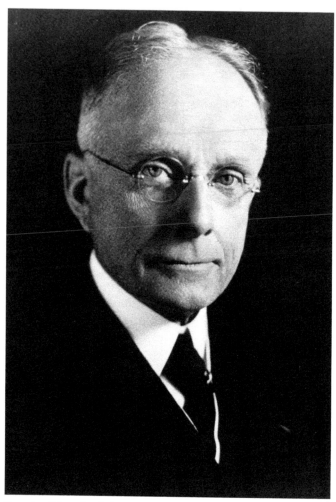

Portrait of Chevalier Jackson. (Credit: Wellcome Library [1].)

82 CHEVALIER JACKSON

Chevalier Jackson (1865–1958) was an American physician and laryngologist. He was one of the founders of modern endoscopy – using tubes to look into the larynx and oesophagus. He published extensively and was a professor at a number of leading American medical schools. An engaging lecturer, he once wrote that 'in teaching the medical student, the primary requisite is to keep him awake' (2). One way to engage students is to use props, and Jackson was a collector of an unusual form of prop. Jackson often performed endoscopies to remove foreign bodies and he kept each of the 2374 inhaled or swallowed bodies that he removed. These included 'buttons, pins, nuts, coins, bones, screws, dentures and bridges, small toys, among many other items' (3). Today, they are housed in the Mutter Museum.

Jackson was known as the father of endoscopy in light of his pioneering work in this field. A curious tradition in medicine and medical education is to bestow the sobriquet 'father of …' a particular specialty on a famous doctor. Examples abound: Cushing as the father of neurosurgery, Halsted the father of modern surgery and, of course, Hippocrates the father of medicine. Is this tradition a literal interpretation of paternalistic tendencies in medical education? Or does the term father suggest a religious figure – who is to be followed and obeyed? Freud was the first to describe the father complex but did not record his thoughts on physicians' penchant for creating father figures. Today, he is called the father of psychoanalysis.

Notes

1. Copyrighted work available under Creative Commons Attribution only licence CC BY 2.0, see http://creativecommons.org/licenses.
2. http://www.philly.com/philly/opinion/20131215_A_pioneer_in_laryngology__he_saved_the_lives_of_many.html (accessed 10 March 2014).
3. http://muttermuseum.org/exhibitions/chevalier-jackson-collection/ (accessed 19 April 2015).

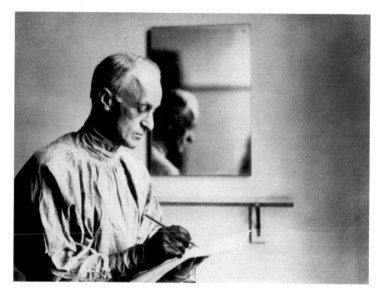

Harvey Williams Cushing. Photograph by W.B. (Credit: Wellcome Library [1].)

83 HARVEY WILLIAMS CUSHING

Harvey Williams Cushing (1869–1939) was an America neurosurgeon and educator. He was the first to describe Cushing's syndrome and the Cushing reflex. His was a life of medical learning and teaching. He developed an interest in science as a schoolboy and learned surgery under the supervision of William Stewart Halsted. After retiring from surgery, he worked as professor of neurology at Yale.

Cushing was a dedicated teacher and an enthusiastic exponent of self-directed learning: 'It is someone's business in every medical school to teach laboratory methods to the students but it is no one's particular business to teach them how to use medical literature …Short talks on the use of the library might well be made an obligatory sectional exercise for students' (2). A surgical aphorism is that a good surgeon knows how to operate and a great surgeon knows when to operate. Cushing was an early advocate of these non-surgical aspects of surgical education: 'I would like to see the day when somebody would be appointed surgeon somewhere who had no hands, for the operative part is the least part of the work' (3).

It is interesting that this photo shows Cushing and his image in the mirror, as by some accounts he was a Jekyll and Hyde character. Cushing was a hard task master and, although dedicated to his patients, was extremely demanding of his residents. According to Lichterman, he 'was charming and selfish, sentimental and racist, devoted to patients and sadistic to his residents, arch-Victorian in his cultural habits and ultramodern in clinical practice, and addicted to work and tobacco' (4).

Notes

1. Copyrighted work available under Creative Commons Attribution only licence CC BY 4.0, http://creativecommons.org/licenses/by/4.0/.

2. Cushing H. Bookshelf browsing: The doctor and his books. *Am J Surg* 1928;4(1):100–110.

3. Letter to Dr. Henry Christian, 20 November 1911.

4. http://www.bmj.com/content/333/7565/451?tab=response-form (accessed 20 April 2015).

MEDICAL EDUCATION
IN THE
UNITED STATES AND CANADA

A REPORT TO
THE CARNEGIE FOUNDATION
FOR THE ADVANCEMENT OF TEACHING

BY
ABRAHAM FLEXNER

WITH AN INTRODUCTION BY
HENRY S. PRITCHETT
PRESIDENT OF THE FOUNDATION

BULLETIN NUMBER FOUR

576 FIFTH AVENUE
NEW YORK CITY

(Credit: Wellcome Library [1].)

84 THE FLEXNER REPORT

Abraham Flexner (1866–1959) was an educationalist and reformer. More than a theoretician, he was keen to test his ideas in the real world and set up his own school shortly after graduating from university. The school enabled learning that was tailored to the needs of the individual and encouraged interactive participation in small groups. The school was a success, and Flexner quickly became an authority in innovative methods of education. He was commissioned to evaluate medical education in North America, and in 1910, he published the Flexner Report – which was to have a revolutionary effect on medical education in North America and worldwide. Indeed, it was to set the landscape for medical education for the new century. The report led to the closure of many rural medical schools and wholesale reform of the practice of medical education. Flexner questioned many traditional aspects of medical education and challenged physicians to justify their practice in teaching. He once asked 'what sound reason can be given for requiring the able and the less able, the industrious and the less industrious, to complete practically the same course of instruction in the same period of time?' (2).

The image shows what Flexner will always be remembered for – the simply and aptly titled *Medical Education in the United States and Canada. A Report to the Carnegie Foundation for the Advancement of Teaching*.

Notes

1. Copyrighted work available under Creative Commons Attribution only licence CC BY 2.0, see http://creativecommons.org/licenses/by/2.0/.
2. Flexner A. Medical education, 1909–1924. *JAMA*. 1924;82(11):833–838.

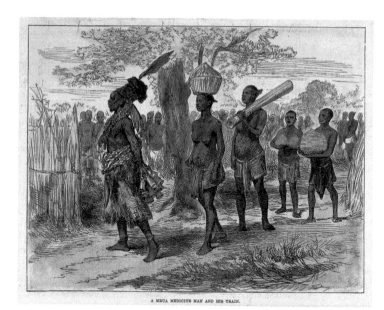

A MRUA MEDICINE MAN AND HIS TRAIN.

A Mrua medicine man or shaman with his assistants, Central Africa. Coloured wood engraving after a sketch by Lieutenant Cameron. (Credit: Wellcome Library [1].)

85 A MRUA MEDICINE MAN, OR SHAMAN, WITH HIS ASSISTANTS

Here is a Mrua medicine man with his assistants. The role of the medicine man was to provide care and to pass on his expertise. The striking feature of the image is not how different it is to Western medical education, but how similar. So the person in command leads from the front, the senior assistants follow close behind and the juniors trail along. All have various instruments to carry. A crowd looks on eagerly – but from a distance. With a different dress code, they could quite easily pass for the consultant surgeon (or chief of surgery), the senior and junior registrars, and the house officers.

What was the learning experience of the Mrua assistants? Perhaps not too dissimilar from the experience of medical students in England in the nineteenth century. According to Edward Thompson writing in 1882, 'it is not enough for a student to have the opportunity of following his teacher round the wards of a hospital, a unit in a hundred or a hundred and fifty others, poking his nose over his comrade's shoulder, and standing upon tiptoe to try and get a glance at what is going on at the bedside of the patient, that the desired end is to be attained' (2).

Notes

1. Copyrighted work available under Creative Commons Attribution only licence CC BY 2.0, see http://creativecommons.org/licenses/by/2.0/.
2. Thompson EC. Address on the past, present, and future of medicine. *BMJ* 1882;2:607.

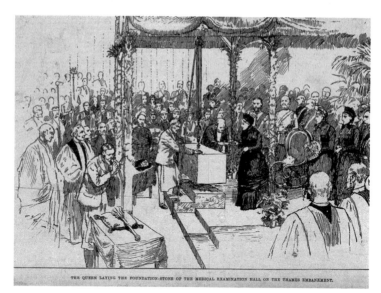

THE QUEEN LAYING THE FOUNDATION-STONE OF THE MEDICAL EXAMINATION HALL ON THE THAMES EMBANKMENT.

The examination hall of the Colleges of Physicians and Surgeons: Queen Victoria laying the foundation stone. Wood engraving. Published: London, 1886. (Credit: Wellcome Library [1].)

86 THE EXAMINATION HALL OF THE COLLEGES OF PHYSICIANS AND SURGEONS: QUEEN VICTORIA LAYING THE FOUNDATION STONE

Medical examinations in the nineteenth century were in much need of reform. Towards the end of the century, Andrew Clark claimed that 'the mere process of cramming conducted by a clever coach may sharpen some of the lower intellectual powers; but it will sap the strength of the higher ones, and, whilst it may carry a student triumphantly through some difficult examination, which may have been made the end of his studies, it will place him in after years at a terrible disadvantage in dealing with the difficult problem of life and work' (2). Twenty years later, James Barr stated that 'mere examining corporations which have done practically nothing for medical education, and are chiefly engaged in extracting fees from students, should be allowed to retire into obscurity' (3).

The process of reform of examinations was to take far longer than was necessary. Indeed examples of poor practice were to continue into the twenty-first century. However, at the time of this engraving, the colleges were certainly starting to reform. They undoubtedly took the task seriously: at the ceremony, they have supplied a weighty stone, atmosphere and monarch.

Notes

1. Copyrighted work available under Creative Commons Attribution only licence CC BY 2.0, see http://creativecommons.org/licenses/by/2.0/.
2. Clark A. An Address on Medical Education and the Duty of the Community with Regard to it. *BMJ* 1888;2:747.
3. Barr J. President's Address, delivered at the eightieth annual meeting of the British Medical Association. *BMJ* 1912;2:157.

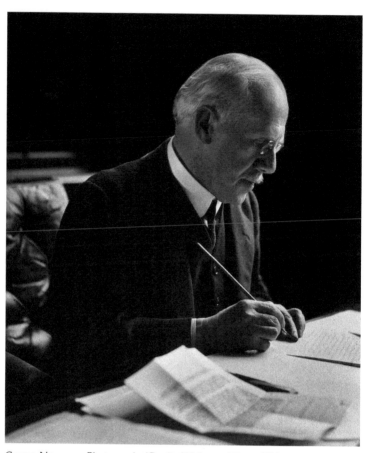

George Newman. Photograph. (Credit: Wellcome Library [1].)

87 GEORGE NEWMAN

George Newman (1870–1948) was a public health physician and England's first chief medical officer. He championed the standardisation of medical education and the education of general practitioners. His thoughts on the importance of medical teachers? 'In short the teacher in a university is the pivot of the method. He must be learned in his subject, skilled in craft, competent in administration, experienced in research, and catholic in mind. He should reach his post not by favour, by merit of age or seniority, by social convention, but chiefly because he is a teacher and a leader of men' (2).

This posed and formal portrait tells us little about Newman the person but a lot about our vision of management and leadership in the first half of the twentieth century. Bespectacled, collared and waist-coated, Newman pores over a desk full of papers, pencil in hand, as if ready to make corrections. Meticulous attention to detail is clearly required for the task in hand. Apart from a leather armchair, the background is invisible – suggesting a man apart from his surroundings. Lastly the leader is alone – perhaps contributing to the concept of the cult of the leader as individual. This concept lingers, even though we all know that everything important happens in teams.

Notes

1. Copyrighted work available under Creative Commons Attribution only licence CC BY 2.0, see http://creativecommons.org/licenses/by/2.0/.

2. Newman G. Some notes on medical education in England. A Memorandum presented to the President of the Board. London, UK: HMSO; 1918, p. 24.

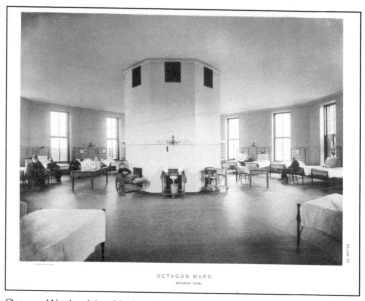

Octagon Ward at Johns Hopkins Hospital – interior. From: Description of the Johns Hopkins Hospital. By: John Shaw Billings. Published: Press of J. Friedenwald, Baltimore, 1890, p. 19. (Credit: Wellcome Library [1].)

88 OCTAGON WARD AT JOHNS HOPKINS HOSPITAL

When physicians and residents visited patients' bedsides on the Octagon Ward, they were said to be doing their 'rounds'. When William Osler led the rounds, they were known as 'grand rounds'. This photograph shows what the ward was like in the absence of both rounds and grand rounds. And the picture is a reasonably healthy one: there is lots of space, the ward is clean, and most importantly patients are dressed and sitting out.

In recent years, there has been growing interest in the learning environment in medical education and the effect that this can have on learners. The context of education is important, and the concept of the learning environment recognises this. The physical aspect of the learning environment matters, but equally important are emotional and social aspects, personal perceptions and organisational aspects and resource and virtual aspects. There is also increasing recognition in medical education that educational provision and clinical care are inextricably interlinked. Education should only be delivered in institutions that provide high-quality care, and learners should be contributing to the delivery of high-quality care from the start of their training. This all requires a variety of skills in educators, including educational and clinical supervision, team-working and the ability to transition junior colleagues from one stage of training to the next.

Note

1. Copyrighted work available under Creative Commons Attribution only licence CC BY 2.0, see http://creativecommons.org/licenses/by/2.0.

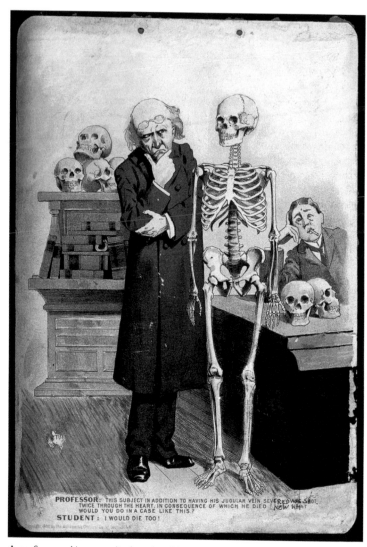

A professor asking a medical student his prognosis for a particular case. Coloured reproduction of a pen drawing. Published: Antikamnia Chemical Co, St Louis, Missouri: 1900. (Credit: Wellcome Library [1].)

89 A PROFESSOR ASKING A MEDICAL STUDENT HIS PROGNOSIS FOR A PARTICULAR CASE

The caption to this picture reads as follows. Professor: 'This subject in addition to having his jugular vein severed was shot twice through the heart, in consequence of which he died. Now what would you do in a case like this?' Student: 'I would die too!' Was this a valid, reliable and fair assessment? Or was it, as Williams would have it, an assessment of 'pedantic learning to gratify the unreasonable demands of insatiable examiners, as Michaelmas geese with piquant seasoning, to suit the depraved tastes of confirmed gourmands'? (2). In his defence, the professor looks too miserly to be a gourmand.

Advances in medical education assessment have meant that scenes such as this are now largely historic. Assessment must be mapped to the curriculum; it must drive best practice in learning and teaching and it must be defensible – with examining authorities being able to show that they have followed due diligence in planning and carrying out the exam (3). Different forms of assessment should be blended together to get a rounded view of the candidate's knowledge, skills and behaviours. So candidates must undergo written, simulation and work-based assessments. Have we lost anything by discarding invalid assessment methods? I think we have lost nothing at all.

Notes

1. Copyrighted work available under Creative Commons Attribution only licence CC BY 2.0, see http://creativecommons.org.

2. Williams WR. Medical education. *BMJ* 1882;2:966.

3. Larsen DP, Butler AC. Test-enhanced learning. In: Walsh K (ed.), *The Oxford Textbook of Medical Education*. Oxford, UK: Oxford University Press; 2013, pp. 443–452.

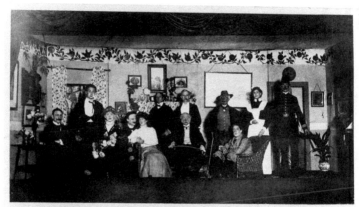

Pinero's 'The New Boy', St. Marys, 1905.

From left to right (all males).

1. Harris, 2. Singer, 3. Brimblecombe, 4. ? Stratom,
5. ? White, 6. Clay (the producer), 7. Mitchell Bird (the
stage manager, standing), 8. Gay-French (sitting down),
9. Zachary Cope, 10. Lascelles, 11. Palmer, 12. Kenneth
Lees.

Members of St Mary's medical school performing 'The new boy'. Photograph.
1905. (Credit: Wellcome Library [1].)

90 MEMBERS OF ST MARY'S MEDICAL SCHOOL PERFORMING 'THE NEW BOY'

Was there ever a golden age of medicine or medical education? When trainees worked 100 hours a week but loved it and still had time to put on a pantomime at Christmas for the patients. I never believed it and was at one with Ezekiel Emanuel when he criticised rose-tinted views of the past: 'At the end of their careers, physicians tend to wax poetic about the art of medicine and how it is being lost. (The same art seems to be lost every generation)' (2). But maybe I have been wrong. Perhaps I should have been reading Chekov rather than Emanuel: 'Medicine is my lawful wife but literature is my mistress. When I am bored with one I spend a night with the other' (3).

In the twentieth century, reforms meant that medicine was seen increasingly as a science and so it slowly lost touch with its roots in the arts and humanities. However, more recently, there has been a rekindling of interest in this link, and so the arts and humanities have a role in today's curricula in many medical schools.

This photograph certainly captures the fun of amateur dramatics – the garish face paint, the outlandish costumes, maybe even some overacting?

Notes

1. Copyrighted work available under Creative Commons Attribution only licence CC BY 2.0, see http://creativecommons.org/licenses/by/2.
2. Emanuel EJ. Changing premed requirements and the medical curriculum. *JAMA* 2006;296(9):1128–1131.
3. Chekhov A. Letter to Suvorin, 1888.

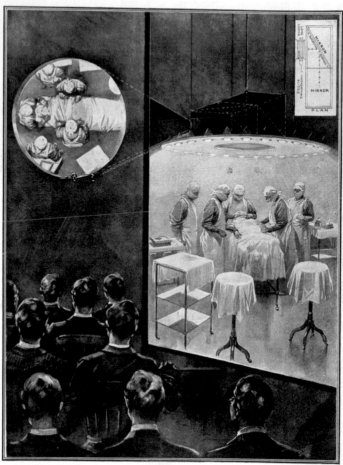

EVERY MOVEMENT OF THE SURGEON SHOWN ON A SCREEN IN THE ROOM NEXT TO THE OPERATING-ROOM.

Medical students observing an operation on a lantern screen via a projecting periscope located above the operating table. Halftone after a drawing by W. Koekkoek, 1909. Published: The illustrated London news, [London]: 17 April 1909. (Credit: Wellcome Library [1].)

91 MEDICAL STUDENTS OBSERVING AN OPERATION ON A LANTERN SCREEN

Technology-enhanced learning in medical education has been with us for over a century. Certainly, the lantern screen enabled students to get an excellent view of the operative field. It worked by means of a projecting periscope located above the operating table. However, it is a moot point as to how much the screen was an advance in educational terms. One is reminded of the aphorism: 'Tell me and I'll forget. Show me and I may not remember. Involve me and I'll understand'. The students were being shown – but were not involved. Ward Griffen put it yet more prosaically: 'you cannot learn surgery sitting on your ass' (2).

Since the days of the lantern screen, much has been done to ensure that medical students are more involved in medicine and surgery and, at the same time, that their involvement is regulated. Legitimate peripheral participation describes the process whereby beginner learners become integrated into a community of practice and eventually develop competence and expertise. At first, involvement is peripheral – learners will participate by means of small and simple tasks that are nonetheless worthwhile. Gradually the learners take on more important tasks and more responsibility until at the end they become core to the process and accepted members of the community of practice.

Notes

1. Copyrighted work available under Creative Commons Attribution only licence CC BY 2.0, see http://creativecommons.org/licenses/by/2.0/.
2. Schein M. *Aphorisms and Quotations for the Surgeon*. Shrewsbury, UK: TFM Publishing Ltd.; 2003, Chapter 28, pp. 68–74.

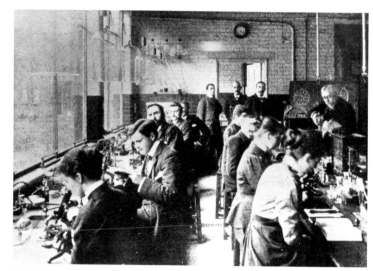

Laboratory at the London School of Tropical Medicine at the Albert Dock Hospital
(Seamen's Hospital Society). 1910. From: Royal Society of Tropical Medicine and
Hygiene. (Credit: Wellcome Library [1].)

92 LABORATORY AT THE LONDON SCHOOL OF TROPICAL MEDICINE AT THE ALBERT DOCK SEAMEN'S HOSPITAL (SEAMEN'S HOSPITAL SOCIETY)

The London School of Tropical Medicine was first located at the Albert Dock Hospital. What better place for teaching and research on tropical medicine than at the point of entry into the United Kingdom? The London School championed education in the medical laboratory sciences, which had sometimes been seen as a Cinderella specialty:

> Why, only last term we sent a man who had never been in a laboratory in his life as a senior Science Master to one of our leading public schools. He came wanting to do private coaching in music. He's doing very well, I believe.
>
> ***Evelyn Waugh (2)***

The London School of Tropical Medicine was founded by Sir Patrick Manson. He felt that there was a need for an institution that could treat people who caught tropical diseases while working in the British Empire. Today the school is located in Gower Street, London, and has become a powerhouse of research and education. It is now known as the London School of Hygiene and Tropical Medicine.

This image shows the laboratory as a hive of activity and learning. The scientists are squinting into microscopes, reading texts, discussing cases with colleagues. Surprisingly there is not a white coat to be seen.

Notes

1. Copyrighted work available under Creative Commons Attribution only licence CC BY 4.0, http://creativecommons.org/licenses/by/4.0/.
2. Waugh E. *Decline and Fall*. Chapman and Hall. 1928.

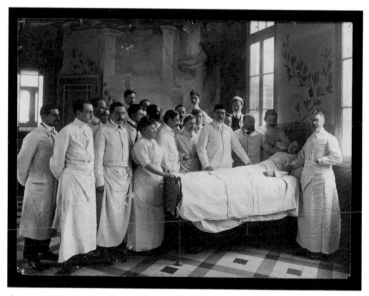

A crowd of medical staff standing round a woman patient in bed in a hospital ward. Murals of foliage and allegories painted on the walls. By: Seeberger Freres. Published: c.1910. Printed: France. (Credit: Wellcome Library [1].)

93 A CROWD OF MEDICAL STAFF STANDING ROUND A WOMAN PATIENT IN BED IN A HOSPITAL WARD

The ward round has been a source of medical learning since the time of Osler. But what is it like for the patient? Certainly, the patient in this photograph seems uncomfortable and worried. Murals of foliage and allegories painted on the walls provide little comfort. The image is reminiscent of Thomas Bernhard's comment on the ward round: 'every day they appeared in front of my bed a white wall of unconcern' (2). There are over 20 people in this wall.

However, since this photograph was taken, much has been done to improve the experience of the patient during teaching ward rounds. Firstly, medical teachers must actively seek and obtain patient consent before taking medical students to see them. Such consent must be freely given, and patients should be empowered to feel comfortable saying no if they do not wish to participate in teaching. Secondly, there has been a move in some quarters to conduct teaching rounds that are separate to the clinical rounds. In this way, the senior clinician can concentrate on teaching – safe in the knowledge that patient care has already been prioritised and dealt with. Thirdly, some patients can deliver medical teaching themselves. Such patients will naturally be intimately familiar with their symptoms and signs and, once trained, can make ideal face to face teachers.

Notes

1. Copyrighted work available under Creative Commons Attribution only licence CC BY 2.0, see http://creativecommons.org/licenses/by/2.0/.
2. Berhard T. Breath – a decision. In: Berhard T (ed.), *Gathering Evidence*. Translated by McLintock, D. New York: Alfred Knopf; 1978/1985, pp. 240–241.

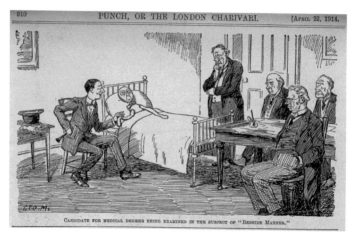

A medical student being examined for his bedside manner by a group of senior doctors. Wood engraving by G. Morrow, 1914. Published: London, 1914. (Credit: Wellcome Library [1].)

94 A MEDICAL STUDENT BEING EXAMINED FOR HIS BEDSIDE MANNER BY A GROUP OF SENIOR DOCTORS

> A difficulty for the current generation of communication skills teachers is that many of us have not had the experience of being formally taught communication skills ourselves.
>
> **Maureen Kelly (2)**

This medical student is being examined for his bedside manner by a group of senior doctors. Teaching and assessing communication skills is a vital duty for the medical educator – yet it is worth pondering the communication skills of this group of examiners. One seems half-asleep, another is looking at the desk, yet another has stuffed his hands deep into his pockets. Only one is actually observing albeit underneath a furred brow and above half-moon spectacles. The patient stares into this distance – his face a mixture of terror and resignation. He has no role in the assessment.

In modern medical education, we would like to think that we are doing better; however, there is still progress to be made. Even in the twenty-first century, all too often, patients have a peripheral role in the assessment of doctors and sometimes their role is little more than tokenism. A better approach would be to ensure patient involvement at a strategic level – in both curriculum design and assessment. In most institutions, there is work to be done before this is achieved.

Notes

1. Copyrighted work available under Creative Commons Attribution only licence CC BY 2.0, see http://creativecommons.org/licenses/by/2.0/.
2. Kelly M. A practical guide for teachers of communication skills: a summary of current approaches to teaching and assessing communication skills. *Educ Prim Care* 2007;18:1–10.

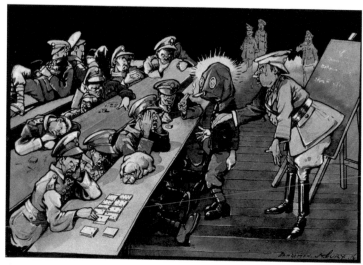

An army officer lectures his bored class on the effects of gas – one student is made to wear a gas mask while another wickedly tries to set light to it. Pen and ink drawing by H. Bury, 1916. (Credit: Wellcome Library [1].)

95 AN ARMY OFFICER LECTURES HIS BORED CLASS ON THE EFFECTS OF GAS – ONE STUDENT IS MADE TO WEAR A GAS MASK WHILE ANOTHER WICKEDLY TRIES TO SET LIGHT TO IT

Few forms of medical education have received such bad press as the lecture. And this image seems to show the lecture in its worst possible form. The class is bored and one student is up to no good. Meanwhile, the rest of the class snooze, yawn and play cards. Even the dog on the front row has fallen asleep.

Modern large-group teaching is more engaging and involves continuous interaction between lecturers and learners. However, it has taken a long time to move on from the practice shown in this image.

Such poor examples of education would no doubt have precipitated this diatribe against lectures from Virginia Woolf: 'Why lecture? Why be lectured? Why, since printing presses have been invented these many centuries, should he [the lecturer] not have printed his lecture instead of speaking it?... Why continue an obsolete custom, which not merely wastes time and temper, but incites the most debased of human passions – vanity, ostentation, self-assertion and the desire to convert? Why encourage your elders to turn themselves into prigs and prophets, when they are ordinary men and women? Why not abolish prigs and prophets?' (2).

Notes

1. Copyrighted work available under Creative Commons Attribution only licence CC BY 4.0, http://creativecommons.org/licenses/by/4.0/.
2. Woolf V. Why? In: *The Death of the Moth*. London, UK: Hogarth Press; 1942.

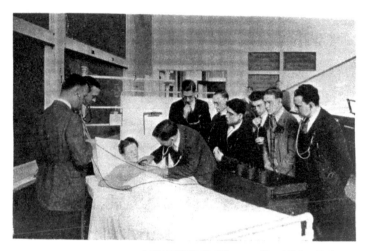

A BEDSIDE DEMONSTRATION. [*General Photographic Agency.*]

A bedside demonstration of the collective stethoscope. From: Heartbeats by Radio. A new use for wireless. The hospital and health review. Published: 1924. New series volume 3, p. 272. (Credit: Wellcome Library [1].)

96 A BEDSIDE DEMONSTRATION OF THE COLLECTIVE STETHOSCOPE

This is another example of technology-enhanced learning from the early twentieth century. This particular device has not stood the test of time. It is worth reflecting on this apparatus and indeed on all new technologies as to whether it is the education that is driving the technology or the technology that is driving the education. New technology is certainly seductive and there is always the temptation to make an extra investment to have the latest high technology and high-fidelity equipment. More thought should probably be given to the cost and value of such investment (2). Value can be increased by ensuring better usage and by aligning institutional investments in technology with the curriculum of the institution.

However, the one advantage of the collective stethoscope is that it must have made the following scenario outlined by Martial rather less of a problem.

> Well, you came, Symmachus, but you brought 100 medical students with you.
> One hundred ice-cold hands poked and jabbed me.
> I didn't have a fever, Symmachus, when I called you – but now I do. (3)

Notes

1. Copyrighted work available under Creative Commons Attribution only licence CC BY 2.0, see http://creativecommons.org/licenses.

2. Ker J, Hogg G, Maran N. Cost-effective simulation. In: Walsh K (ed.), *Cost Effectiveness in Medical Education*. 2010, pp. 61–71, Radcliffe, Abingdon.

3. http://www.bookdrum.com/books/tom-jones/183034/bookmark/193014.htmlb (accessed 10 March 2014).

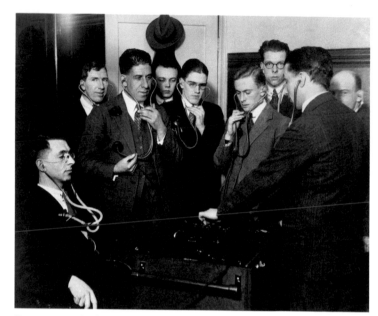

Doctors or medical students listening to their heartbeats using a multiple stethoscope. Photograph, 1920s. By: Central News. (Credit: Wellcome Library [1].)

97 DOCTORS OR MEDICAL STUDENTS LISTENING TO THEIR HEARTBEATS USING A MULTIPLE STETHOSCOPE

This is yet another example of technology-enhanced learning. In the absence of high-resolution imaging of the heart, auscultation was a vital skill to be learned by repeated practice. Once again, it is worth considering the balance between educational and technological advances. This is a consideration that must come to the fore when any new technology is used in medical education. E-learning in medical education is just the latest example of this (2). According to Sandars, 'the potential for e-learning can only be achieved if an approach is used that concentrates on the education and recognises that the role of technology is to enhance the learning, rather than trying to find educational uses for new technology' (3).

This photograph signifies concentration – the learners are looking in different directions but all are listening intently. It is also interesting to see how medical students dressed in the early part of the twentieth century. This exclusively male group are all wearing suits, collars and ties. This uniform was not worn for clinical reasons; however, it likely reinforced the image of the doctor as a learned gentleman. Today, infection control teams ensure that ties are dispensed with and that arms are bare below the elbow. In turn, some complain that doctors now look too informal. However, they probably look more approachable, and that is in keeping with the fashion of the times.

Notes

1. Copyrighted work available under Creative Commons Attribution only licence CC BY 2.0, see http://creativecommons.org/licenses/by/2.0/.

2. Walsh K. Online educational tools to improve the knowledge of primary care professionals in infectious diseases. *Educ Health* 2008; 21(1):64.

3. Sandars J. What is e-learning? In: J Sandars (ed.), *E-Learning for GP Educators*. Oxon, UK: Radcliffe Publishing; 2006, pp. 1–5.

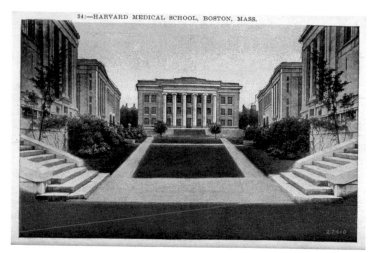

34:—HARVARD MEDICAL SCHOOL, BOSTON, MASS.

Postcard of Harvard Medical School, Boston, United States. Photograph, 1928. (Credit: Wellcome Library [1].)

Harvard Medical School is one of the oldest medical schools in the United States. It was founded in 1782 by John Warren, Benjamin Waterhouse and Aaron Dexter. Notable alumni include Oliver Wendell Holmes Senior, Harvey Cushing and Atul Gawande. Harvard has always encouraged a spirit of freedom and enquiry amongst its students and faculty, and in the twenty-first century Gawande is leading the way. He has written on the imperfect science of medicine and surgery, on surgical performance and on the importance of planning and organisation in healthcare.

One of the chapters in Gawande's book *Complications* is entitled 'Education of a Knife'. Here, Gawande gives a vivid insight into the mind of the learner surgeon. He describes the anxieties, fears and doubts of the learner, which are slowly replaced by competence and confidence (but never arrogance). The emotions of learning have traditionally been neglected in medical education; however, we ignore these emotions at our peril.

According to Larry Wall, Harvard also encourages a spirit of freedom and enquiry amongst its microorganisms: 'The Harvard Law states: Under controlled conditions of light, temperature, humidity, and nutrition, the organism will do as it damn well pleases' (2).

This image shows the school in all its glory on Longwood Avenue. Does the 'Great White Quadrangle' against the background of an azure sky capture the sacredness of medicine and medical education? Or is it all just too much?

Notes

1. Copyrighted work available under Creative Commons Attribution only licence CC BY 2.0, see http://creativecommons.org/licenses/by/2.
2. http://www.searchquotes.com/quotation/The_Harvard_Law_states:_Under_controlled_conditions_of_light,_temperature,_humidity,_and_nutrition,_/241772/ (accessed 10 March 2014).

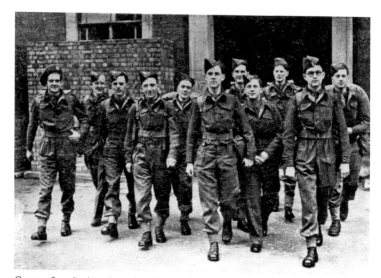

Group of medical students from Westminster Hospital who worked at Belsen
after its liberation by the Allies. Photograph, 1945. From: Papers of Major Allen
Percival Prior: Photographs of the personnel involved with the aid to inmates
of Belsen Concentration Camp... including photographs of the inmates and
treatment. Collection: Archives & Manuscripts. Library reference no.: Archives
and Manuscripts RAMC 1801/1/6. (Credit: The RAMC Muniment Collection in
the care of the Wellcome Library, Wellcome Images [1].)

99 GROUP OF MEDICAL STUDENTS FROM WESTMINSTER HOSPITAL WHO WORKED AT BELSEN AFTER ITS LIBERATION BY THE ALLIES

Belsen concentration camp was liberated by the allies in 1945 and soon afterwards medical students from the United Kingdom came to work there to help the many thousands of ill and starving inmates. Initial attempts to help inmates of concentration camps often went wrong. Prisoners were fed too much too quickly – this caused the 'refeeding syndrome' – and many died as a result of biochemical electrolyte disturbances caused by their rescuers' well-meaning efforts. However, army medics learned from their initial mistakes, and education, on how best to care for people with severe malnutrition quickly spread amongst allied armies.

But these fresh-faced recruits will hopefully have learned more than just biochemistry as a result of their experiences. Many years later, Polly Toynbee wrote that 'it is in the nature of every profession to set itself an ideal character and attempt to impose it as best it can on new entrants. It is also in the nature of humanity to fail that ideal most of the time' (2). In this case, however, the medical students are certainly trying to live up to this ideal character. Their faces wear expressions that we would hope to see in any group of medical students – determination, concern, purpose; some of them are even smiling.

Notes

1. Copyrighted work available under Creative Commons Attribution only licence CC BY 4.0, http://creativecommons.org/licenses/by/4.0.
2. Toynbee P. Between aspiration and reality. *BMJ* 2002;325:718.

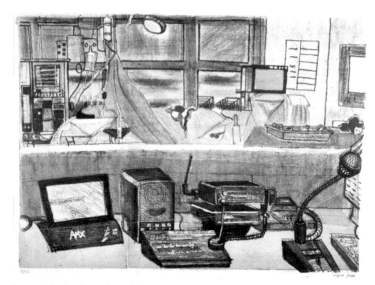

The Eagle simulator for training anaesthesia students at the Chelsea and
Westminster Hospital, London. Etching with lithograph by Virgina Powell, 2000.
(Credit: Wellcome Library [1].)

100 THE EAGLE SIMULATOR FOR TRAINING ANAESTHESIA STUDENTS AT THE CHELSEA AND WESTMINSTER HOSPITAL, LONDON

This is the Eagle simulator used for training anaesthesia students at the Chelsea and Westminster Hospital. Simulation has many natural advantages in medical education: it enables learners to practice clinical and communication skills and to integrate those skills; it enables them to practise and rehearse as often as they like; it enables them to practice in interdisciplinary teams. According to Ian Curran, the 'huge benefit of simulation is that it shifts the steep and dangerous part of the learning curve away from patients' (2). Simulation also enables learners to practice their skills in a learning environment that is safe for themselves as well as for patients.

This is the most modern image in the book and yet it is already starting to look old. Perhaps it is the sketchy futuristic style that makes it look dated. Or perhaps it is the pace of change in simulation and technology over the past 15 years. It is easy to forget that mobile technology was still in its infancy at the turn of the century. What does it tell us about the future? The only certainty is that the pace of change will continue for some time to come.

Notes

1. Copyrighted work available under Creative Commons Attribution only licence CC BY 2.0, see http://creativecommons.org/licenses/by/2.0/.
2. Reynolds T, Kong ML. Shifting the learning curve. *BMJ* 2010;341:c6260.

INDEX

T - #0850 - 101024 - C234 - 198/129/10 - PB - 9781498751964 - Gloss Lamination